HARMONY
by DESIGN
Navigating Work and Life in Healthcare

Sharon M. Weinstein, MS, RN, CRNI-R®, CVP, CSP, FAAN

Marla J. Vannucci, PhD

Katie Boston-Leary, PhD, MBA, MHA, RN, NEA-BC, FADLN, FAONL

Foreword by Jean Watson

Sigma
GLOBAL NURSING
EXCELLENCE

Sigma Theta Tau International Honor Society of Nursing (Sigma) is a nonprofit organization whose mission is developing nurse leaders anywhere to improve healthcare everywhere. Founded in 1922, Sigma has more than 85,000 active members in over 100 countries and territories. Members include practicing nurses, instructors, researchers, policymakers, entrepreneurs, and others. Sigma's more than 600 chapters are located at more than 700 institutions of higher education throughout Armenia, Australia, Botswana, Brazil, Canada, Chile, Colombia, Croatia, England, Eswatini, Finland, Ghana, Hong Kong, Ireland, Israel, Italy, Jamaica, Japan, Jordan, Kenya, Lebanon, Malawi, Mexico, the Netherlands, Nigeria, Pakistan, Philippines, Portugal, Puerto Rico, Saudi Arabia, Scotland, Singapore, South Africa, South Korea, Spain, Sweden, Taiwan, Tanzania, Thailand, the United States, and Wales. Learn more at www.sigmanursing.org.

Sigma Theta Tau International
550 West North Street
Indianapolis, IN, USA 46202

To request a review copy for course adoption, order additional books, buy in bulk, or purchase for corporate use, contact Sigma Marketplace at 888.654.4968 (US/Canada toll-free), +1.317.687.2256 (International), or solutions@sigmamarketplace.org.

To request author information, or for speaker or other media requests, contact Sigma Marketing at 888.634.7575 (US/Canada toll-free) or +1.317.634.8171 (International).

ISBN: 9781646482108
EPUB ISBN: 9781646482115
PDF ISBN: 9781646482122

PRAISE FOR *HARMONY BY DESIGN: NAVIGATING WORK AND LIFE IN HEALTHCARE*

"Harmony by Design *gets directly at the heart of what it takes to live a meaningful life—purpose, engagement, integration, mindfulness, awareness, and compassion—and it does so in a practical and easy-to-grasp way. The authors masterfully blend the personal with the professional to help the reader understand how to create an overall environment that allows them to find balance. I appreciate that technology-related challenges are addressed explicitly, as this is a critical modality that will only increase in ubiquity and has an undue role in the balance-imbalance dynamic. The authors get an A for developing a framework, tools, and resources that empower our dedicated healthcare colleagues to find the harmony that works for them.*"

–Apurv Gupta, MD, MPH
Vice President, Premier, Inc.

"*An absolute must-read!* Harmony by Design *masterfully redefines work-life harmony. Weinstein, Vannucci, and Boston-Leary take readers on an incredible journey packed with practical tools and profound insights, empowering professionals to conquer burnout and thrive at living their best lives!*"
–Dr. Jason Gleason, DNP, FNP-C, FAANP
USAF Lieutenant Colonel (RET)

"Harmony by Design *provides a comprehensive guide to living a life in harmony with our priorities and values. It is thoughtful, practical, and empowering. What a gift to have the tools to help us find control during these challenging times!*"

–Bonnie Barnes, FAAN
Co-founder, The DAISY Foundation

"*Drs. Marla Vannucci and Katie Boston-Leary, led by Sharon Weinstein, have written an essential guide for healthcare professionals navigating the demands of a challenging industry.* Harmony by Design *goes beyond theory, offering practical tools to achieve work-life harmony and resilience. With actionable strategies and balance brevities, the book empowers readers to align well-being with professional goals, addressing burnout, compassion fatigue, and stress. This is a must-read for anyone seeking harmony amid the complexities of today's healthcare environment. It's a valuable resource for those striving to integrate personal and professional life without compromise.*"

–Renee Thompson, DNP, RN, FAAN, CSP
CEO & Founder, Healthy Workforce Institute

"*As the healthcare workplace undergoes a profound transformation, giving healthcare professionals the tools and insights they need to be at their best on the job has never been more important.* Harmony by Design *initiates and drives an important conversation about work-life harmony and how to engage it at a critical time in healthcare. The result is a more complete way to support and care for healthcare providers so they can better support and care for the rest of us.*"

–Joe Mull, MEd, CSP
Founder of Boss Hero School and Author of *Employalty*

Library of Congress Control Number: 2025027037

Publisher: Dustin Sullivan

Acquisitions Editor: Emily Hatch

Development Editor: Jillmarie Leeper Sycamore

Cover Designer: Rebecca Batchelor

Interior Design/Page Layout: Rebecca Batchelor

Indexer: Larry D. Sweazy

Managing Editor: Carla Hall

Publications Specialist: Todd Lothery

Project Editor: Todd Lothery

Copy Editor: Todd Lothery

Proofreader: Todd Lothery

Illustrator: Kimb Williams

DEDICATION

This book is for you—wherever you are and whatever challenges you face. It stands as a testament to the work we have done in workforce well-being and the work environment for over 25 years. Rooted in collective wisdom from practice, education, and process, *Harmony by Design* reflects the evolving needs of individuals and teams striving for fulfillment in both work and life.

We write this with you in mind, celebrating your remarkable perseverance and dedication to those around you. Our content is aligned with the American Association of Colleges of Nursing *Essentials,* which, while designed for nurses, provide valuable guidance for all professionals seeking to create a workplace and life that values harmony. Many debate whether work-life balance is truly attainable, but perhaps the real goal is harmony or integration. Whatever path you choose, your resilience lights the way for others.

May this book help you cultivate the well-being, fulfillment, and alignment you deserve on your journey ahead.

Fondly,
Sharon, Marla, and Katie

ACKNOWLEDGMENTS

I've been truly blessed with a loving family whose unwavering belief in me—and in my vision to help others unlock their fullest potential—truly matters. As we work to change the world, it's important to remember the everyday human needs of those we touch.

I'm deeply grateful to the two incredible professionals and our contributing author, whose collaboration brought this book to life.

And a heartfelt thank you to my husband, Steve, for always encouraging me to chase my dreams and become the best version of myself. Life is made up of expansive goals and simple, harmonious moments, like spending time with grandchildren, who make each day extraordinary.

Savor those moments!

S. M. W.

Thank you to the team of professionals from Sigma, including Emily Hatch, Acquisitions Editor; Carla Hall, Managing Editor; Todd Lothery, Project Editor, Copy Editor, and Proofreader; Jillmarie Leeper Sycamore, Development Editor; Rebecca Batchelor, Designer; and Larry D. Sweazy, Indexer. We thank Kimb Williams, Graphic Designer, for her creative approach and whose vision brought our ideas to life. And, finally, thanks to the co-authors, Drs. Marla J. Vannucci and Katie Boston-Leary, and contributing author Dr. Monica Holliday, each of whom has found harmony in their life and communicates the model each and every day. They now share their message with you, the reading audience. These are lessons learned from those who have lived them.

The author team, led by Sharon M. Weinstein, brings together the unique talents and wellness insights of three experienced leaders. With diverse expertise in practice, process, workforce dynamics, workplace culture, psychology, and education, they offer a fresh perspective on achieving harmony in today's world. Read on . . . it's within your reach!

About the Authors

Sharon M. Weinstein, MS, RN, CRNI-R®, CVP, CSP, FAAN, is the CEO of SMW Group LLC, partner at Diagnostic Think LLC, Chair at the HBA Ambassador Learning Center Impact Workshops, and the American Nurses Enterprise Innovation Community Manager. Her 40-year career blends executive leadership, clinical practice, and education. An award-winning author of 25 books and 170+ articles, she's also a frequent podcast guest

Known as the "Stressbuster," Weinstein is all about helping people handle the pressures of today's fast-paced world. She shares practical strategies to manage stress and crises, whether at work or in personal life. Inspired by design thinking, her fresh take on stress management is helping organizations improve engagement, boost productivity, and build healthier workplace cultures. Weinstein knows how to navigate the blurred lines between work and life, equipping people with the tools they need for harmony.

Weinstein is passionate about helping professionals find success and happiness without burning out. Through her commitment to education, work/life balance, and workplace wellness, she's impacted lives in over 50 countries.

Weinstein was pivotal in founding Sigma Theta Tau International's first chapter in Armenia. Adjunct faculty at the University of Illinois Chicago and Purdue University Global, her research focuses on caregiver well-being and workplace culture. A Past President of the National Speakers Association (NSA)-DC and Past Chair of the Certified Speaking Professional Committee of NSA, her contributions have earned her numerous accolades, including Fellow of the American Academy of Nursing, the John J. Daly Award for Outstanding Service and Chair's Award for Distinguished Service from the National Speakers Association, the Outstanding Performance Award from the Infusion Nurses Society, the Frist Humanitarian Award from the Hospital Corporation of America, and the People's Choice Award from TEDx UStreet.

She rode a camel in Cairo, was a delegate to the Women's Conference in Beijing, designed the foreign patient department at the Kremlin Hospital in Moscow (yes, that Kremlin), and has been featured in and on *CEO Magazine, The Globe and Mail, The Washington Post, Crain's Chicago Business, Enterprising Women, HuffPost, Forbes, The Chicago Tribune,* NBC, and TEDx. Sharon's commitment is simple: "Infuse health and reduce stress," making the workplace better for everyone.

Marla J. Vannucci, PhD, has spent over 25 years helping healthcare professionals, educators, veterans, parents, and families navigate life's challenges, from managing stress and trauma to finding balance during transitions. She is the owner and Executive Director of Blue Sage Psychotherapy Group PLLC and an Adjunct Professor in Adler University's

Clinical Psychology program. Previously, she served as an Associate Professor of Psychology for 13 years at Adler University, where she earned recognition for her research on mentorship, employee training, and wellness.

Vannucci has authored articles for consumer-focused and peer-reviewed publications about stress and trauma, compassion fatigue, nursing, and clinical training issues. She has extensively provided education and training programs to healthcare personnel and other helping professionals. Previously, she was the Director of Clinical Services at the Chicago School of Professional Psychology, where she coordinated mental health services for students and served as Training Director for pre- and post-graduate clinical training programs. Before this role, she was a Senior Consultant at Deloitte Touche Tohmatsu, where she specialized in working with healthcare organizations, designing consumer-focused wellness programs, providing leadership training, improving workflows, and implementing employee performance and development systems. Her expertise has been featured on WBEZ, Mom Talk Radio, and in publications like *The Economist, The Washington Post,* OncologyTimes.com, and *HuffPost.*

Beyond her clinical and scholarly endeavors, Vannucci is a musician and voting member of the Recording Academy. She writes and performs "kindie" (kids' indie) music that promotes social-emotional learning and healthy expression while providing entertainment for families to enjoy together. Her "kindie" releases earned a Mom's Choice Gold Media Award (2022) and a Creative Child Magazine Award (2023) and have been featured nationally and internationally on children's radio and in educational programs. Vannucci was a contributor to *B Is for Balance,* 2nd edition, and we welcome her to the writing team of *Harmony by Design* as a co-author.

Katie Boston-Leary, PhD, MBA, MHA, RN, NEA-BC, FADLN, FAONL, is the Senior Vice President of Equity and Engagement at the American Nurses Enterprise. Best known for her work in nursing practice, work environment, and Healthy Nurse/Healthy Nation, she is an Adjunct Professor at the University of Maryland School of Nursing and the School of Nursing at Case Western Reserve University. She is a board member for St. John's University Health Programs, Hippocratic AI, and Ingenovis Health and editorial advisory boards with Nursing Management, Nursing 2023, and ACHE.

Boston-Leary's impact goes even further—she serves on the National Commission to Address Racism in Nursing. She works with the National Academies of Sciences, Engineering, and Medicine's National Plan to Address Clinician Well-Being, supported by the US Surgeon General, Dr. Vivek Murthy. She authored two chapters—"Social Justice" and "Advocacy"—in the *Sage Encyclopedia of Multicultural Counseling, Social Justice, and Advocacy,* the first encyclopedia focused on racism and diversity, equity, inclusion, and belonging. She was also featured in the documentary film *Everybody's Work,* produced by SHIFT Nursing and funded by the Robert Wood Johnson Foundation.

As a key player in solving the nurse staffing crisis, Boston-Leary led a National Nurse Staffing Think Tank and Task Force, which published actionable recommendations to address the nurse staffing crisis. She is also a 2024 International Council of Nurses Global Nurse Leadership Institute Scholar. She testified on panels and roundtables on Capitol Hill on the nurse staffing crisis and regulatory burden on hospitals and nurses. She also serves as a faculty member for the Institute for Healthcare Improvement's Health Equity Program for senior leaders.

Boston-Leary was named one of HealthLeaders Media's "Five Chief Nursing Officers Changing Healthcare" and won several awards, including the 2023 ICABA TD Bank Woman of Impact and the 2024 Spectrum Circle Award for Innovation in Health. She's a Distinguished Fellow with the Academy of Diversity Leaders in Nursing and the National Black Nurses Association.

Her research with major organizations like Quint Studer, Joslin Insight, and McKinsey, and her national and international speaking engagements, make her a well-known voice in the field. You might have seen her in *Forbes, Beckers,* CNBC, *the New York Times, Bloomberg News,* or NBC's *Today Show,* where she discussed the ongoing nurse staffing crisis. Her thought leadership continues to influence the conversation on staffing, diversity, and the future of healthcare.

Contributing Author

Monica Holliday, PsyD, is a clinical psychologist with over 15 years of experience helping adolescents, adults, and families enhance positive communication, improve household climate, and support transitions through key life changes, including helping those who have experienced significant loss process their grief and move forward. She earned her doctorate in clinical psychology from Adler University with a concentration in childhood and adolescence. Her expertise with children and families comes from her work providing community and school-based training and consultation to parents and providing clinical services in community mental health, therapeutic day school, an attention and learning disorders clinic, and private practice. As a certified Positive Discipline Parenting and Classroom Educator, she has developed an evidence-based approach to positive discipline, a popular parenting program. Her research on parent self-efficacy was recently published in the peer-reviewed journal *Individual Psychology.* In her work with parents, Holliday advocates for a balanced approach to family life, where boundaries and nurturance are equally emphasized. Her research illuminates how this approach— which incorporates mutually respectful communication—reduces stress, increases connection, and builds confidence in both parents and children. She also serves as an Adjunct Professor at Adler University, training the next generation of psychologists in proven methods to better support parents and families.

ADDITIONAL BOOK RESOURCE

A *Learning Guide and Workbook* for this book is available for sale from most retailers. Ask your bookseller or simply search for this book title with added keywords of "learning guide" or "workbook" to purchase it. You can also email our Marketplace team for bulk orders at solutions@sigmamarketplace.org.

SPECIAL NOTE TO READERS

Here at Sigma, we realize that language is constantly evolving. The meaning of a word often changes over time, some words become obsolete, and some terms that were once acceptable may become controversial or even offensive, depending on the context or circumstances. We have made every effort to make language choices that are inclusive and not offensive. Should you identify words in this book that you believe negatively impact a group or groups of people, please reach out to us at Publications@SigmaNursing.org.

B truly is for balance,
a harmony of health and grace.
We invite you to embrace it,
in every moment, every space.

May you care for yourselves,
and for one another too,
with the same passion, the same heart,
that you give to all you do.

For every voice and every role,
in the workforce, far and near,
let the same devotion guide you,
and bring balance, calm, and cheer.

Self-care is not selfish,
it's the key to being whole—
nurture body, mind, and spirit,
to renew and heal your soul.

—Sharon M. Weinstein

TABLE OF CONTENTS

FOREWORD

Harmony by Design goes beyond the concept of balance, inviting a deeper sense of connection—both within ourselves and across the many dimensions of our lives. This work builds upon Sharon Weinstein's original foundation of balance, evolving into a powerful guide for harmonized living, mental well-being, and the creation of healthy work environments. It delivers a message that both inspires and equips individuals to navigate the seemingly impossible demands of daily life with greater ease and intention.

Weinstein and co-authors Marla J. Vannucci and Katie Boston-Leary remind us that rather than striving for perfection, we can embrace the harmony found within life's imperfections. Through grace, compassion, care, and patience, they offer a framework to help us cope with imbalance and unrealistic expectations while fostering a more sustainable and fulfilling way of living and working.

What makes *Harmony by Design* strikingly unique is its alignment with the latest Essential Competencies from the American Association of Colleges of Nursing. In a world where maintaining harmony can feel elusive, this book provides actionable steps for integrating personal well-being with professional growth. It outlines 10 competency-based strategies, serving as a road map for both personal reflection and professional development, guiding readers toward a more intentional, fulfilling, and harmonious life. They include, for example, specific strategies for:

- Engaging meaningfully with life and work as one integrated whole

- Navigating technology and social media with mindfulness

- Staying aware of and prioritizing your mental health

- Building resilience and managing stress effectively

- Striving for work/life integration rather than just balance

- Embracing compassion as a guiding principle in daily life

The authors guide readers through key aspects of life, including reflecting on life's purpose, confronting our humanity and inner doubts with intention, acknowledging the illusion of control, addressing compassion during fatigue and stress, and facing failures and risks beyond our comfort zones. These dynamic vicissitudes of our human existence are grounded in core values and embrace all life experiences.

The work extends beyond negotiating strategies for harmonized living into personal and organizational responsibility. It translates reflective, insightful change into creating a supportive, healthy work environment. This section raises a new level of conscious attention to personal responsibility and what may be framed as relational accountability—being in the right relationship with oneself and others. It invites readers to develop as informed leaders who foster a caring community of belonging and trust.

Contemporary and pressing futuristic topics are addressed, such as information overload and its long-term effects. The book explores how to face these challenges mindfully, set healthy digital boundaries, and implement personal and professional action steps. It stands as a comprehensive, guided resource for deep change from within to face life holistically, beyond a "balance mentality." This work invites the reader into the future, considering further personal and professional growth, including coaching for career advancement and pathways toward becoming the best version of oneself. It helps readers discover their passion, ideals, and vision, creating a blueprint for what lies ahead.

Finally, *Harmony by Design* transcends "balance" per se. It extends into an invitation to engage in concrete philosophical and strategic steps toward living a fulfilled life of authentic coherence. In turn, this work serves as a foundational resource and guide for realigning oneself in personal and professional harmony. It helps readers cultivate and sustain a meaningful connection with their evolving selves, grounded in compassion, reflection, and core values, while transforming personal growth into authentic, harmonized leadership. Anyone at any stage of their career, including nurses and those working in health-related fields, can grow and evolve through the content, wisdom, and concrete, experiential, and existential guidance of this book, using it as a tool for personal evolution and meaningful leadership.

–Jean Watson, Watson Caring Science Institute

PREFACE: A NEW EVOLUTION BUILDING ON
B IS FOR BALANCE

In the delightful words of Mary Poppins:

> *"For a spoonful of sugar helps the medicine go down.*
> *The medicine go down, the medicine go down.*
> *Just a spoonful of sugar helps the medicine go down.*
> *In a most delightful way."*

But my wise colleague, Dr. Bernadette M. Melnyk, offers a slightly different prescription. She suggests that while sugar might make medicine easier to swallow, the best way to sweeten your day is with a daily dose of Vitamin G—for gratitude!

Unlike sugar, Vitamin G has no side effects, calories, or limit on its benefits. Starting each morning with a grateful heart can boost your mood, strengthen your resilience, and add a delightful shine to even the cloudiest day.

So tomorrow morning, skip the spoon.

We often treat our professional and personal lives as separate, but in reality, we have one life, and the balance we seek reflects our inner state. *Harmony by Design* prioritizes cultivating harmony over chasing balance, recognizing that fulfillment comes from integrating all aspects of life.

This book is for professionals, multitaskers, and leaders striving to be everything to everyone. It introduces an innovative approach, applying design thinking to life-work harmony. Rather than viewing balance as a fixed goal, this perspective encourages a dynamic, evolving process.

The hallmark predecessor to this book, *B Is for Balance,* explored foundational concepts of work-life balance and then introduced 12 key steps, including engagement, sleep health, and longevity. *Harmony by Design,* enriched by Drs. Marla J. Vannucci and Katie Boston-Leary and contributor Monica Holliday, offers a fresh path to achieving a more sustainable and fulfilling life.

As someone who has reinvented herself throughout her career, I've seen firsthand how elusive harmony can be. Yet, despite my success, I often found that harmony was absent, and the cost of that imbalance was too high, especially when it came to family relationships. The pandemic blurred work-life boundaries, forcing many to juggle remote work, return to office, caregiving, and home responsibilities. Some families grew closer, while others faced stress due to increased time together (too much of a good thing). Work-life harmony became a struggle for many, affecting mental health.

My 13-year-old granddaughter said it best:

"School is good because it keeps me socially active. When I had COVID, I started talking to the walls."

–Julia L. Weinstein
Holton-Arms School

How many of us have felt that way?

Thank you, Marla, Katie, and Monica!

–Sharon

INTRODUCTION

For years, we have sought balance and turned to various resources for guidance. Now, we're proud to introduce *Harmony by Design: Navigating Work and Life in Healthcare*. Three expert co-authors offer fresh insights, practical tools, and new perspectives. This book goes beyond the concept of balance, exploring harmony, resilience, and sustainable career strategies in today's evolving world. With real-world applications and actionable strategies, *Harmony by Design* empowers professionals to cultivate well-being, effectiveness, and fulfillment in both their work and personal lives. Harmony is achieved by intentionally designing a fulfilling life where each element supports the whole, fostering a sense of wholeness rather than rigid balance. This book offers a practical road map for integrating personal and professional life with purpose and intention, creating a foundation for long-term success and fulfillment.

Harmony by Design is a powerful, stand-alone manual offering innovative strategies to navigate today's complex challenges. Whether used on its own or alongside the *Learning Guide and Workbook*, it provides practical examples, actionable insights, and a clear path to lasting success—no matter your role or contribution. If you're ready to lead the road to harmony with intention and impact, this is for you.

HOW TO USE THIS BOOK

Harmony by Design shifts the focus from rigid balance to work-life integration, aligning with the American Association of Colleges of Nursing *Essentials* for professional nursing. This playbook offers valuable tips, tools, and strategies to enhance job satisfaction, reduce burnout, and foster a harmonious lifestyle. Organized into five parts, it provides 10 competency-aligned strategies with actionable insights for achieving balance in both personal and professional life. Harmony arises not from perfection but from fluidly honoring each part of life, creating space for growth, alignment, and fulfillment. This approach empowers readers to navigate the complexities of their roles while maintaining well-being and purpose.

Use this book as your road map, with guidance on:

- Engaging meaningfully in life and work
- Navigating technology and social media mindfully
- Building resilience and managing stress effectively
- Achieving work/life integration, not just balance

Each section is structured to provide insight and practical steps you can apply immediately, helping you build a rewarding career and life.

Elements in the Book

The "Designing Harmony" boxes provide exercises to help you visualize and categorize the various demands in your life, providing a clear framework to assess areas that need more attention or adjustment. They are designed to integrate harmony into daily life.

The "Finding Balance" and "Harmony Reflection" boxes offer a deeper exploration of thought-provoking insights and prompts for self-discovery.

The "Balance Brevities" are quick, actionable exercises designed to be brief yet impactful, offering immediate steps you can take to restore or maintain balance in your day-to-day routine. You will find them again at the start of each chapter in the accompanying *Learning Guide and Workbook*, along with a "how-to" tool for implementation.

Each tool serves a unique purpose in helping you achieve and sustain harmony, from broad assessments to focused, practical strategies.

Resources and References

At the end of each chapter, you will find a curated list of resources and references for further reading, providing additional avenues to explore specific topics in greater depth. These references include scholarly articles, books, and other authoritative materials that will support your learning and offer broader perspectives on the concepts discussed.

Whether you're just beginning your career or looking to advance, these references will serve as valuable tools to guide your journey. Expect to find materials that not only align with your professional goals but also focus on fostering personal well-being, helping you create a holistic approach to success and fulfillment.

I

UNDERSTANDING AND APPRECIATING SELF

1

DISCOVER YOUR PURPOSE

Marla J. Vannucci, PhD

The question of why we are here has been asked for as long as humans have been on our planet. You may value connectedness to others, growth and learning, or making the world a better place. You may find meaning in spirituality or faith—or you may value all of these. Because you are reading this book, you are very likely invested in helping others. And if you focus significant energy on helping others, then it is also probably true that your needs rarely reach the top of your priority list. Homing in on what is most meaningful allows you to define your purpose. This chapter provides tools to define your purpose and use it as a "North Star" for balance in your life.

WHY ASK WHY?

One of my patients often found himself in the role of rescuer. He referred to himself as the "go-to guy." He could always be counted on for a ticket to a big concert, a shoulder to cry on, or even to save someone from a dangerous situation. He was the fixer, the one people called when in need. However, over the years, he struggled to identify what should be central in his life. We often discussed how the rescuer role, while rewarding, can be a lonely path. True fulfillment as a helper, I explained, requires mutuality, where the call to respond deeply nourishes us—where we give and receive.

When he later stepped in to help raise his friend's son, he reevaluated his life choices. He even changed his career goals to spend more time with the child, who began to call him "Dad." But when his friend and her son moved abroad with her new partner, my patient was devastated. He feared he would be replaced in his son's life and struggled with the sense of loss. Through reflection, he realized that his connection wasn't about the title of "Dad" but about being a consistent and loving presence for his son. What drove him was a calling, not an obligation, and he learned that being in the father role benefited both his son and himself.

His journey eventually led him to become a special education teacher, where he found a profound sense of purpose. Helping others was no longer about fixing problems; instead, it meant forming meaningful connections with students, mentoring and guiding them. He learned that purpose gives direction to actions and relationships. It empowers and grounds us, connecting us to something greater than ourselves, and guides us to live authentically and intentionally.

Let's explore how you can identify your purpose.

"At the center of your being, you have the answer; you know who you are, and you know what you want."

–Lao Tzu

My patient became a fixer not through intention but because he was good at it. Others sought him out, and he felt obligated to help. He didn't mind the role at first, but it left him feeling unfulfilled and disconnected over time. Once he discovered his true purpose, he transitioned into a more meaningful helper role that aligned with his own goals and needs. However, this shift required him to step outside his comfort zone and try something new. Without purpose, we often rely on overused strengths, hindering growth and flexibility.

Overused strengths have been popularized in leadership development, but therapists have recognized them for decades (Kaiser & Overfield, 2011; McCall, 2009). *Overused strengths* occur when we excessively rely on skills or traits that have been helpful to us, applying them in situations when they are less relevant or less effective. Rather than pushing ourselves to foster underdeveloped skills, especially when we are uncomfortable or in the unfamiliar, we may lean into what we already know and try to make it fit. In fact, we may even confuse overused strengths with purpose, leading us to lean in even further. In these cases, our strengths can become weaknesses, leading to frustration, anxiety, or feelings of powerlessness. In therapy, we often help patients identify overused strengths and help them cultivate lesser used abilities.

As a management consultant for Deloitte Touche Tohmatsu, I coached senior leaders, and I recall one particularly memorable client who was very proud of how he used humor to connect with his team. During a financial downturn, however, his reliance on humor became inappropriate when his employees faced job insecurity. He was unsure how to support his team, and his discomfort led him to continue making jokes, resulting in a human resources complaint.

Overusing strengths leads to rigidity. In contrast, knowing our purpose promotes flexibility, providing a foundation for us to try new things, experiment, and be spontaneous. By defining our purpose, we gain flexibility to respond appropriately to new challenges, and we align our true selves, enabling us to navigate life authentically and with greater ease.

A former patient had always been the responsible, compliant child in a family where her older brother required lifelong care. She struggled with defining her identity and focused on being "perfect," earning straight A's, and acting as a third parent to her brother. This led to social anxiety, isolation, and a lack of meaningful relationships. Therapy helped loosen her rigid view and encouraged her to explore suppressed aspects of her personality, like her great sense of humor. She started to socialize, volunteer, and even took an art class.

Her transformation demonstrated how overused strengths can limit growth. Although she would eventually become her brother's caretaker, this was not her only purpose in life. By broadening her sense of self and embracing her purpose, she could explore new experiences and relationships. Just like bodybuilders who may lack flexibility, we, too, can become rigid when we rely too heavily on our known strengths. Purpose drives behavior beyond external rewards, allowing us to grow, adapt, and embrace vulnerability. When we act from purpose, we can confidently navigate new challenges, knowing that our intention guides us.

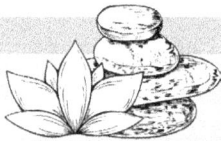

DESIGNING HARMONY EXERCISE 1.1

Reflecting on Your Strengths

Reflect on your personal strengths at work and in your personal life. Identify five strengths, write them down, and consider these questions:

1. Are there experiences in your life that have promoted the development of these specific strengths versus others? What challenges or positive factors in your life required or encouraged these strengths?

2. Are there times that you over-rely on one or more of these strengths to cope, problem-solve, or manage relationships? Why might you do this?

3. Do any of these strengths ever become weaknesses?

4. What would it feel like to try something new in one of these situations? How might you handle the discomfort that arises?

THE PATH TO PURPOSE

Some discover their purpose by accident, stumbling upon what's meaningful through experience. Here we engage in a systematic and deductive process to identify and apply values. We explore a three-step method: values sorting, role-model reflection, and mission-building.

Ask yourself . . .

What gives your life meaning?

SORTING OUT YOUR PURPOSE

Card sorting, also called *Q-sort* or *Q methodology* (betterevaluation.org, 2022; Van Exel et al., 2005), has been used in social sciences research, management and leadership, employee development, career counseling, and psychotherapy to rank or organize values, skills, preferences, feelings, experiences, or ideas (Brown, 1993; Stephenson, 1953). This technique groups or categorizes concepts to understand the relationships among ideas. When working with couples, I might ask them first to independently rank what they value most in a relationship and then compare their lists, reflecting on how the similarities and differences contribute to conflict or connection. As a management consultant, I used card sorting to help clients identify the most critical skills in a job and then apply the results to construct a targeted recruitment strategy and interview protocol to find qualified candidates.

Values sorting is a great way to discover what is most important in your life. A quick search online reveals many sorting tools, including app-based and online options described below. These digital tools do not provide "blank cards" for customizing, so I've included instructions on how to do this. The "analog" tool shared here combines elements from my favorites. Additional resources, including physical card sets for use in team-building, can be found at the chapter's end and in the Appendix. The exercise that follows walks you through using a values card sort to identify your "Core Five" values, which represent elements of your purpose and the foundation for achieving greater alignment and harmony.

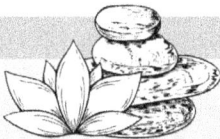

DESIGNING HARMONY EXERCISE 1.2

"Core Five": Sorting Your Values

Note: If you prefer to complete this exercise digitally, use the provided links under Resources at the end of this chapter to select a digital tool. Before using the tool, review the 60 words provided below to identify any missing from the online tool. After you complete the online tool using their instructions, go to Step 7 to compare and adjust your finalists.

Step 1: Table 1.1 lists 60 values with definitions. Write each word on a single Post-it note, or make a copy of the two pages from this text and cut the boxes into evenly sized "cards."

Step 2: Review the definitions to determine if you agree with the wording provided. You might think about one of the words differently or dislike part of the definition. Feel free to write your updated definition on your Post-it note or card. Or, if you own the copy of the book you are holding, feel free to write on this page.

Step 3: Are any words missing from the list that are important to you? If so, add those words to Post-its or make additional cards. Also remember to write down your definitions.

Step 4: Lay the cards on a table or stick them to the wall so that you can see them all. Keep the list with definitions below handy if you need to reference it.

Step 5: Take three blank Post-its/cards and label them as "Absolutely Critical," "Important," and "Less or Not Important." Place them on the wall or table to create three areas for sorting.

Step 6: Consider the importance of each value in your *ideal or preferred life.* Currently you may not be living your most valued values, whether due to inadequate resources, confidence, awareness, or support. You will identify these issues later and create a plan to address them. For now, focus on what would be most important to you without barriers. Sort an even number of cards into each category. Work quickly and follow your first instinct.

Step 7: Review your choices to ensure you have categorized correctly and make any changes. Put the "Important" and "Less or Not Important" piles aside. Now, re-sort the "Absolutely Critical" pile to narrow it down to the top five cards. (If you completed this task using a digital tool, bring out the words you added to compare them to the finalists from the digital tool.) One way to narrow down to five is to compare two cards to each other at a time. For example, hold Autonomy in one hand, and one at a time, compare the other cards in your "Absolutely Critical" pile to Autonomy. For example, which is more important, Compassion or Autonomy? The winner stays in the pile. Then, compare the loser to the next card. Any card that wins stays in the pile, and each time, the loser is compared to the rest. If you end with more than five cards, start again with the surviving cards, and do this as many times as needed to get to the top five. Keep in mind as you eliminate cards that you do not have to eliminate these values from your life. We are simply ranking and prioritizing to get to the most foundational.

Step 8: Review the final five. How do you feel about selecting these as the Core Five? Are they core to how you think about yourself, your relationships, and who you are in the world?

Step 9: Congratulate yourself on completing the values sort and finding your Core Five.

TABLE 1.1 Value Words Chart

Certainty	Comfort	Perseverance	Discipline	Loyalty	Harmony
Order, predictability	Feeling or putting others at ease	Hard work, a finisher	Routine, structure	Dedication, commitment	Calm, grounded, balanced
Health	**Meaningful work**	**Growth**	**Family**	**Influence**	**Variety**
Attending to physical fitness, caring for mental and physical health	Meaningful activities, a positive impact	Lifelong learning, intellectual, emotional, or spiritual development	Spending time with family members	Being a role model, impacting others' decisions	Change, novelty
Compassion	**Creativity**	**Stability**	**Autonomy**	**Justice**	**Integrity**
Caring for others, kindness toward others and oneself	Innovation, inventiveness, artistry	Sufficient finances, freedom from worry about resources	Making choices, directing one's own behavior/ work	Fairness, equality	Honesty, quality, following a code of conduct, ethics
Spirituality	**Security**	**Freedom**	**Privacy**	**Excellence**	**Intimacy**
Intangible aspects of life, spiritual experiences	Freedom from danger or threat	Liberty, freedom of thought and action	Time by yourself, discretion	Mastery, striving for high performance	Connections with others, friendship, sharing thoughts and feelings
Peace	**Collaboration**	**Pleasure**	**Ambition**	**Achievement**	**Competence**
Freedom from conflict	Sharing ideas, teamwork, compromising	Enjoyable or satisfying experiences, personal gratification	Desire to succeed and go further in career	Attaining goals, productivity, industry	Developing skill, expertise, abilities
Trust	**Recognition**	**Reputation**	**Power**	**Independence**	**Wisdom**
Trusting others and being trustworthy	Valued and honored by others, fame	Perceived by others in a positive way	Making decisions for others, having authority, being in charge	Self-reliance, self-sufficiency	Knowledge from experience, making good decisions

continues

TABLE 1.1 Value Words Chart (cont.)

Flexibility	Teaching	Tradition	Status	Uniqueness	Community
Adapting, going with the flow	Sharing knowledge, mentorship, developing others	Customs, rituals, history and culture, conforming to norms	Reaching a specific level or role of significance	Defining yourself, doing what is true to you	Belonging to a group, connecting to others, contributing to building community
Happiness	**Challenge**	**Adventure**	**Wealth**	**Contribution**	**Courage**
Contentment, joy	Testing abilities, pushing yourself, competition	Exploration, trying new things	Obtaining money, material items, luxury	Helping others, service, philanthropy	Bravery, persisting in the face of risk/danger
Advocacy	**Beauty**	**Caring**	**Fun**	**Accountability**	**Diversity**
Standing up for your own and others' rights, being assertive	Aesthetics, appreciation of beauty, creating or cultivating beauty	Caring for others, the environment, or a cause	Enjoying yourself, having fun, humor, laughter, playfulness	Responsibility, dependability	Acceptance and tolerance of differences, celebrating differences
Reason	**Passion**	**Intuition**	**Authenticity**	**Efficiency**	**Relaxation**
Logic, problem-solving	Doing what you love, immersion	Following instincts, going with your gut	Staying true to what matters, being the real you	Not wasting time, planning	Leisure, rest breaks, self-care

(Adapted from the Center for Ethical Leadership, 2002; Harris, 2010)

ENACTING THE "CORE FIVE"

Branding expert Brian Sooy defines purpose in an organization as the company's reason for being—*why* it exists (Sooy, 2013). *What* will be done to realize or fulfill that purpose is referred to as *vision*. And the steps taken to put that vision into action—or *how* the vision comes to fruition—is the organization's *mission* (Choy, 2021). To put your purpose into action, you must also answer *why*, *what*, and *how*. Your Core Five is your *why*. Now that you know your Core Five, the next step is to determine *what* you will do

Ask yourself . . .
What do you notice as the main themes in your life?

to enact the Core Five and *how* you will accomplish this. One way to do this is to observe others who share your values and reflect on how they live these values.

HEROES AND ROLE MODELS

Many of us have come to our values by watching others, such as parents, grandparents, other relatives, teachers, friends, neighbors, or spiritual leaders. Some may identify "heroes," real or imaginary, who are role models for our values. Joseph Serrano, artist-in-residence at the Theraplay Institute and a licensed mental health clinician in private practice (and my former student), is a leading researcher on comic book characters' emotional and moral impact. In an email to me dated November 19, 2024, Dr. Serrano explained:

> Numerous studies illustrate the impact of role models in one's life, regardless if these individuals are real or fictional. In the world of comic books, stereotypical "heroes" traditionally advocate selflessness, service to others, a level of conscience, and an awareness of consequences in order to attain a moral life. Conversely, perceived "villains" tend to illustrate qualities of self-centeredness, hunger for power, a sense of entitlement, lack of care, and sinisterness that typically lean towards an immoral life. While the distinction between the title of "hero" and "villain" is relative to the viewer's perspective, these role models can offer a point of reference for goals, standards and values, and behavioral tendencies.

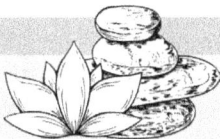

DESIGNING HARMONY EXERCISE 1.3

Heroes and Role Models

We learn values both from positive and less positive role models, whether real people or fictional characters. Keeping in mind your Core Five, consider the following questions. It may be helpful to use a piece of paper divided into five columns, one for each of the Core Five, to capture your responses, or you can combine several values into a single set of responses. Note that a sample appears in the *Learning Guide and Workbook*.

Think about someone whom you associate with this value:

- What do you recall about the first time you observed this value in this person? What was memorable?
- What did/do they do that demonstrates this value?
- How did you feel?
- Which specific behaviors or characteristics of theirs would you like to emulate?

- Which strengths or abilities did they use?
- What can you learn from this to help you enact your values?

Now, think about yourself.

- What in your own actions, behaviors, or attitudes reflects this key person?
- What are your current strengths, skills, abilities, passions, or interests that align with or support living this value? How can you apply them to living this value?
- What are your vulnerabilities or gaps in skills that make it hard to live this value?
- What do you need to know, understand, realize, do, feel, think, or experience to support living with this value?
- What can you do to obtain the skills or knowledge you need to live this value?
- What are the barriers or obstacles that exist right now?
- What can you control, or what can you impact?
- Who can help you overcome obstacles, and what resources do you need? How can you ask for help from this person?

Your Mission if You Choose to Accept It

Putting your purpose into action can be depicted by an equation:

Purpose Action Plan = Why (values) + What (vision) + How (goals, objectives, mission) + Who

For your plan to be actionable, your target audience(s) must be identified, as well as how you might fulfill your vision with that audience. The following exercise will help you describe your target audiences, as well as how you will impact them by enacting your Core Five.

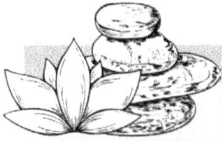

The Who, What, and How Chart

This activity helps organize variables related to living your values. Create a table with headings listing potential audiences, such as family, self, or community, using Table 1.2 as a guide.

TABLE 1.2 The Who, What, and How Chart

	My Sample	Your Plan
The Target Audience	Professional community	
Actions (what you will do to serve/impact this audience)	Create an educational platform for healthcare professionals	
Values (values enacted)	Teaching, stability, meaningful work	
Tools (existing strengths, skills, knowledge, resources)	Public speaking, teaching experience, ideas and content for courses, professional network, creativity, expertise in subject matter areas	
Needs (needed skills, knowledge, resources, support)	Time and energy to complete continuing education sponsor application, partner to share the workload, technology platform, mentor who has done this before, consultation from accountant for pricing, expand my professional network	
Next Steps (what you can do now or in the next four weeks; how can you get started/gain momentum?)	Set aside three hours weekly to develop the platform; identify who could be a mentor and partner and contact them	

Now you can use the Who, What, and How Chart to develop your Purpose Action Plan. Follow these steps:

1. Start with the Next Steps identified in Exercise 1.4. How will you put these into action to feel immediate momentum?

2. What skills or resources do you need to enact your plan? Create a realistic timeline to develop the skills, access the resources, or gain buy-in from potential partners.

3. Reflect on how you will leverage your tools without over-relying on strengths.

4. Now lay out your master plan—again, the timeline should be realistic. Allow for breaks in the action to rest, reflect, and reassess. How is the plan going? What needs to be adjusted moving forward?

Getting to Balance: Aligning Your Purpose

Your Purpose Action Plan helps you live intentionally and authentically by defining who you want to be across situations. Enacting your purpose brings consistency in your attitudes and behaviors, clarifying what matters most. Knowing your purpose means being value-driven, and balance comes from staying true to those values, regardless of the setting. While learning from differences is essential for growth, misalignment of your values with those of your organization, supervisor, community, friends, or even your family can create internal conflict, which increases your risk for significant stress, burnout, and even mental health concerns.

Work-Life Alignment

The concept of work-life alignment suggests that balance comes from aligning our core values and true selves across different roles and settings and not from achieving some ideal distribution of work and personal tasks and activities. Stress and anxiety can arise when we are forced to hide our true selves or behave in ways inconsistent with our values. At its extreme, role conflict occurs when our actions contradict our core beliefs.

A personal example highlights this issue: I once taught in a graduate program focused on community-based interventions driven by social justice and systemic change. However, during an economic downturn, the program merged with a for-profit entity, promising to maintain its values. Over time, corporate culture overshadowed our original mission, and the staff became increasingly disillusioned. The program's mission statement was replaced with one focused on corporate goals, and many staff members, including myself, left due to the misalignment of values.

This type of misalignment is a common source of role conflict. In healthcare, for instance, the daily challenges of role ambiguity and conflicting expectations lead to burnout, stress, and poor job performance. These issues, in turn, jeopardize patient care. Addressing these concerns requires aligning organizational values with the well-being of employees. A key question remains: Do your values align with those of your employer or organization?

CONGRUENCE

Organizational change may take time, but congruence can help manage the disparity among personal and organizational values and role challenges. Carl Rogers defined *congruence* as the alignment between one's ideal self and actual experience (Rogers, 1961). When my patients struggle to feel this alignment, I call it "living in the gap"—they can feel stuck in the space between who they want to be and how they spend their time right now. Knowing your purpose is key to congruence, as it serves as a guiding "North Star" for self-concept and behavior—knowing your *why* helps you know *what* to do and *how* to do it. Living intentionally in alignment with our purpose across different settings makes us more grounded and connected.

Ask yourself . . .

What is the "essence" of you? How does your essence show up across different situations, relationships, or experiences?

Does this essence matter for the question "What gives my life meaning?" Why or why not?

What types of activities take up most of your day? Do they reflect your essence or who you are at the core?

What contribution do you want to make? How does that contribution fit with your essence?

BALANCE BREVITIES . . . ACTION STEPS

Here are six tips you can take on the road to balance:

1. Identify your overused strengths.

2. Make a plan to strengthen an underused asset or ability.

3. Sort your Core Five.

4. Identify a hero or role model.

5. Assess your work/life values alignment.

6. Do something today congruent with your purpose.

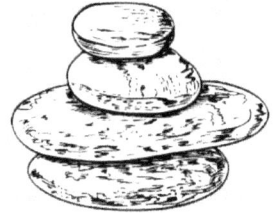

RESOURCES

Digital Card Sorting Tools

Vantage Core Values Exercise app (iOS & Google): App-based tool for sorting core values. https://apps.apple.com/us/app/core-values-exercise/id1590790024

Online Values Card Sort (if you would like to use this tool for the Core Five exercise, stop after you have selected five values rather than narrowing it to three): https://www. bridgehopefamilytherapy.com/values-exercise/

Physical Card Sets

Veeken Values Card Set (John Veeken): https://www.cavershambooksellers.com/search/9780980517538

Other Purpose & Mission Resources

Sinek, S., Mead, D., & Docker, P. (2017). *Find your why: A practical guide for discovering purpose for you and your team*. Penguin Random House.

REFERENCES

betterevaluation.org. (2022). *Q-methodology*. https://www.betterevaluation.org/methods-approaches/methods/q-methodology

Brown, S. R. (1993, January). A primer on Q methodology. *Operant Subjectivity, 16*(3/4), 91–138. http://dx.doi.org/10.22488/okstate.93.100504

Center for Ethical Leadership. (2002). *Self-guided core values assessment.* https://www.ethicalleadership.org/uploads/2/6/2/6/26265761/1.4_core_values_exercise.pdf

Choy, E. K. (2021, Oct. 17). How to find your work's purpose through storytelling. *Forbes.* https://www.forbes.com/sites/estherchoy/2021/10/17/how-to-find-your-works-purpose-through-storytelling/

Harris, R. (2010). *A quick look at your values.* https://www.actmindfully.com.au/wp-content/uploads/2019/07/Values_Checklist_-_Russ_Harris.pdf

Kaiser, R., & Overfield, D. (2011). Strengths, strengths overused, and lopsided leadership. *Consulting Psychology Journal: Practice and Research, 63*(2), 89–109. https://doi.org/10.1037/a0024470

McCall, M. W., Jr. (2009). Every strength a weakness and other caveats. In R. B. Kaiser (Ed.), *The perils of accentuating the positive* (pp. 41–56). Hogan Press.

Rogers, C. R. (1961). *On becoming a person: A therapist's view of psychotherapy.* Houghton Mifflin.

Sooy, B. (2013, Nov. 22). *The difference between purpose, mission, and vision.* Aespire.com. https://www.aespire.com/blog/communications/the-difference-between-your-purpose-and-mission

Stephenson, W. (1953). *The study of behavior: Q-technique and its methodology.* University of Chicago Press.

Van Exel, N., Job, A., & de Graaf, G. (2005). *Q methodology: A sneak preview.*

"The past, the present and the future are really one: they are today."

–Harriet Beecher Stowe

2

EMBRACE ENGAGEMENT IN YOUR LIFE

Marla J. Vannucci, PhD

Everyone has spaced out while driving, lost in thought, only to arrive at their destination without fully realizing it. When we operate on autopilot, we miss opportunities for creativity, joy, purpose, and balance that come from greater engagement.

What Is Engagement?

In my work as a clinical psychologist, many of my patients with depression describe feeling as though they are in a fog. One patient said, "I feel like I can't touch my life, as if I'm in a cloud." While this sense of disconnection is common in depression, it's not exclusive to it. People with seasonal allergies, ADHD, anxiety, PTSD, burnout, or sleep disorders may also experience similar fog-like sensations that disrupt daily life. In today's fast-paced world, life often feels like a never-ending to-do list rather than a meaningful experience. Engagement is key to overcoming this feeling.

In this chapter I explore two types of engagement: mindful engagement, which involves focused attention and intentionality in the present, and flow, where one becomes fully absorbed in an activity.

Mindfulness Grows Your Capacity to Change

Mindfulness is not a new concept. While its roots are in Buddhism, Jon Kabat-Zinn is often credited with bringing mindfulness into Western conversations (Nash, 2019). Practicing mindfulness can be an emotional and spiritual experience, but the scientist in me appreciates the underlying biochemistry that leads to feelings of well-being in the short term and cognitive and emotional flexibility in the long term. As a biological process, today's mindful engagement helps you right now, and consistent mindful engagement helps you even more later.

Studies link mindfulness to better immune functioning (Davidson et al., 2003), and reduction in symptoms of anxiety disorders (Kabat-Zinn et al., 1992) and major depression (Galante et al., 2013). Additionally, mindfulness practice is associated with improved psychosocial functioning in those struggling with chronic somatic illnesses, such as cancer (Bohlmeijer et al., 2010; Ledesma & Kumano, 2009); better management of binge eating behavior (Kristeller & Wolever, 2011); and reductions in daily stress and job burnout (Flook et al, 2013; Goodman & Schorling, 2012; Williams et al., 2001).

Through mindfulness, you can change your brain, allowing you to feel calmer, be more aware of yourself and your life, have a greater sense of control, and make better choices that will help you reach your goals.

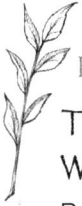

The Morning Snuggle: Engagement as the Entry Point to Well-Being

Before becoming a mother, I struggled to be in the moment, always juggling countless "to-dos." After my son was born, I realized I needed to push myself to focus solely on him in order to truly care for him. The early years were filled with anxiety. Was he safe? Was he eating enough? Once I returned to work, I made time each morning for a "morning snuggle" with him in our rocker, treating it like daily meditation. I reminded myself, "These moments won't last forever." Instead of rushing, I allowed myself to be present, which brought peace and joy. Now that he's 16, it's easy to forget to be fully present as he talks about his interests. Yet, every Sunday, we grab mugs of coffee and explore country backroads together. We sing to the radio, and sometimes, he shares details of his teenage world. These moments of engagement bring me happiness, connection, and meaning.

ASSESSING YOUR ENGAGEMENT

- Think about moments in your life when you feel happiness or satisfaction. What are you doing? Are you alone or with others?

- How engaged are you in your life right now? Are there moments where you are fully present and in the moment?

- Is there a challenging activity at work or in your life in which you become completely immersed and do not notice time pass? How do you feel when engaged in this task?

If you imagine that engagement is a coin, the two sides of that coin are experiences of acute, in-the-moment self-awareness and losing oneself in deep immersion. These are the two types of engagement that promote well-being.

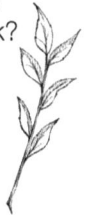

PRACTICING MINDFULNESS

Mindfulness practice can be formal, like meditating or participating in a mindfulness-based stress reduction program, or informal, such as eating lunch or folding laundry mindfully. All mindfulness practice involves three elements: intention, attention, and attitudes (Shapiro et al., 2006). *Intention* means actively deciding to be present—intention alone can shift us out of autopilot. *Attention* refers to consciously focusing on a specific task, while also noticing or observing your experience of that task. Lastly, Kabat-Zinn (2013) identifies nine mindful *attitudes* that help us recognize and challenge unhelpful and typically automatic thought patterns. While we can benefit from practicing all nine attitudes, we can likely identify a handful that are the hardest to overcome and need the most practice. A complete list of the attitudes is in the *Learning Guide and Workbook*, but I will share a few here that are particularly beneficial for helping professionals.

Mindful Attitudes

The *beginner's mind* involves letting go of preconceived notions and approaching situations with fresh eyes as if experiencing them for the first time. Young children practice the beginner's mind every day, as they notice things adults overlook, like hearing a bird sing or feeling sand for the first time. I remember when my son saw a bird for the first time, and it made me realize that I no longer paid attention to the birds around me. This awareness of disconnecting from nature reminded me to stop and notice the world again. Try this: Select a part of your morning routine and pretend that this is the first time you have ever brushed your teeth, cooked breakfast, or put gas in the car. What do you notice in approaching the task for the first time?

The *non-striving* attitude encourages us to let go of our constant need to achieve. Many of us are so goal-oriented that we miss the present moment. Try this: Throughout your day, see if you can catch yourself thinking about the outcome of a task and redirect yourself to focus on the activity itself. How does it feel to make this shift?

Non-judgment invites us to observe our thoughts and actions without labeling them as good or bad. We may not even notice the evaluative messages playing in the background of our minds as we go about our daily business, deciding if what we just said or did is OK, and often similarly assessing those around us. The brain can jump to conclusions because it likes shortcuts, and we may decide how we feel about what someone else is saying before they even get a full sentence out. Try this: Throughout your day, notice if you automatically make judgments about what people are saying and doing, including yourself. Are you able to redirect your energy instead to hold curiosity? Ask questions to learn more.

Practicing these mindful attitudes enhances openness, creativity, and cognitive flexibility, leading to improved problem-solving, a greater capacity to manage stress, and overall well-being. See the *Learning Guide and Workbook* for two additional beginner's mind exercises and a description of all nine mindful attitudes.

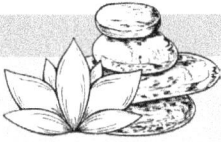

Everyday Mindfulness

Informal mindfulness practice is intentionally finding moments throughout the day to turn your attention to what you are doing and experience it more fully. Try bringing intention, attention, and mindful attitudes to these everyday moments:

- **Morning routine:** While showering or brushing your teeth, pause and notice if you are planning for the day rather than noticing scents, sensations, and sounds.

- **Walking:** Notice your thoughts and body positioning. Move your shoulder blades back and relax. Refocus on your body and notice your breathing and movement.

- **Interacting with others:** Listen with intention. Experience verbal and nonverbal cues and notice yourself listening.

- **Mindful check-in:** Use a phone or tablet app to remind yourself to be mindful. For 60 seconds, notice your internal experience. What is your mood? How does your body feel? Return to your activity with greater presence.

Meditation

Meditation is a tool for formal mindfulness practice that can range from five minutes to much longer sessions. Like any practice, beginning with smaller increments and building up over time is important. Key aspects include breathing, body awareness, posture, refocusing wandering thoughts, and paying attention to sensations and feelings. Yoga is another mindfulness practice. Experimenting with different styles helps you find what works best. Guided meditations and resources are provided at the end of this chapter. What follows is a simple five-minute meditation.

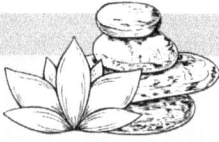

Five-Minute Meditation

Five minutes of meditation is enough to face the day with presence and engagement. Find a comfortable place to sit or lie down. Rest your hands at your sides. If you find that you fall asleep while lying down during this exercise, then try sitting instead. Close your eyes if you wish.

Notice your breath entering and leaving your body. It may feel cool entering and warmer as it leaves. Notice the rhythm of your breath and how your chest expands and falls as the breath enters and leaves. How does your breathing sound? What sensations are there?

Your mind will likely wander. Notice these thoughts without judgment or reactivity and then refocus on your breathing. Tell yourself that you are present in this moment and that you have nowhere else to be. Set a reminder on your phone or computer to tell you when the five-minute practice time has passed.

Congratulate yourself for giving yourself this time to practice.

Adapted from Stahl & Goldstein, 2019

"Happiness is absorption."

–T. E. Lawrence, diplomat and writer

FLOW

Now, let's explore the concept of flow, the other side of the engagement coin. While mindfulness enhances present-moment awareness, *flow* occurs when we lose ourselves in an absorbing task. In this state, self-awareness fades, and deep immersion takes over. Often referred to as "being in the zone," the flow experience will actually be interrupted and hindered by intentional focus and attending to self-awareness (Csikszentmihalyi, 2008). We usually notice when we're unhappy but rarely notice when we're happy—because we're fully immersed in the moment (Kral & Idlout, 2012). In flow, we focus on the activity, not our inner thoughts (Huskey, 2022).

ELEMENTS OF FLOW

Flow activities are intrinsically rewarding and usually involve some type of immediate feedback. Flow at work means focusing on the task's challenge or appeal rather than the paycheck or our assessment of our performance. Flow requires a balance of skill and challenge—tasks shouldn't be too easy or too difficult. A too-easy task will bore us, and a too-difficult task will require focus and attention that will hinder flow or create frustration. When an activity aligns with our skills and challenges us just enough, we have clear goals and a loss of self-consciousness; we are in the "sweet spot" of flow (Csikszentmihalyi, 2008; Jackson & Eklund, 2012). Flow can occur in physical activities like running or cycling and even sedentary tasks like reading. At work and home, distractions unfortunately often interrupt flow.

THE SCIENCE OF FLOW

The neuroscience of flow is still evolving. Research shows that flow is linked to decreased activity in brain areas related to self-focus and executive functions and greater activity in regions tied to goal orientation and the dopaminergic reward system (van der Linden et al., 2021). Activation of the reward system contributes to feelings of optimism, energy, and motivation and could explain the experiences of intrinsic motivation, commitment, focus, and happiness in flow. Flow promotes well-being (Wu et al., 2021), even under stress (Sweeny et al., 2020), and can act as a mediator in the relationship between technology use and well-being (Huskey, 2022; Shao et al., 2024). Flow also fosters resilience (Tabibnia, 2020) and protects against burnout and depression (Aust et al., 2022).

FLOW IN BALANCE

Flow is a state of harmony, where attention and immersion, effort and outcome, and investment and reward are in balance. We experience synchronicity between mind and body, with reduced self-monitoring and stress. This state promotes relaxation and a sense of capability. Many report experiencing flow at work, and those who do tend to have higher job satisfaction and commitment, leading to better retention (Maeran & Cangiano, 2013). However, overwhelm can hinder flow, as unrealistic workloads may create challenges that prevent flow, even when skills match the task. Healthcare professionals experiencing workplace bullying or discrimination may face diminished flow as well. Once thought to be discrete, flow is now seen as a continuum. We can increase flow by aiming for more frequent, longer, or more intense experiences, as well as modifying environmental factors that hinder it (Bartholomeyczik et al., 2023).

ENHANCING FLOW

Once we understand what makes flow experiences unique, we can create strategies to enhance flow in our daily lives:

- Add a goal or challenge. Add meaning or passion. Do something in your life that matters to you, even if for a brief period. Before mundane tasks, remind yourself of their importance.

- Eliminate interruptions. Set a timer to keep others at bay, or if you can't, find ways to include others in your task—then give them a challenge.

- Improve your skills. More skills means more activities that can become flow. Are there opportunities to specialize that you can pursue?

- Let go of the inner critic. Self-consciousness hinders flow, so focus more on the task and less on observing yourself.

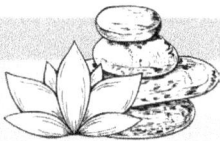

DESIGNING HARMONY EXERCISE 2.3

Assessing Flow

Does your job hit the "sweet spot" in balancing skill and challenge? When do you feel a sense of obligation? Where can you incorporate elements of flow?

EXERCISE

Label one side of a piece of paper "work" and the other side "personal." On each side, create two columns labeled "stress" and "boredom." For "stress," write down ideas for how you can promote flow by decreasing the stress associated with tasks—such as ways to increase skill, decrease self-criticism, reduce distractions, or collaborate with others. Under "boredom," identify strategies to make tasks more meaningful—set a goal, increase the challenge, reprioritize, find where your passion lies, or highlight the task's importance.

Compare your "work" and "personal." Where are there more opportunities for flow? If at work, you may run the risk of workaholism. If at home, you may experience deep dissatisfaction with your job. Identify one strategy you can implement right now and decide how you will take action. To implement your strategy, do you need to increase the challenge or increase your skill?

Flow increases well-being and happiness at work and in our personal lives. Look for ways to balance skill and challenge to manage stress, experience greater meaning, and find your flow "sweet spot."

"True life is lived when tiny changes occur."
–Leo Tolstoy

ENGAGEMENT AND FLEXIBILITY

Have you ever gone to work despite being sick? Many view this as a badge of honor, but showing up without being mentally present is an example of disengagement that disrupts balance. This phenomenon, called *presenteeism*, occurs when individuals work while physically or mentally unwell, often due to job insecurity, financial concerns, or internal pressures like perfectionism and guilt (Chander et al., 2023). We may also resort to presenteeism because we hold rigid ideas about meeting others' or our own expectations, and we may not allow ourselves the flexibility to make a different choice. Organizations can also promote presenteeism through understaffing and excessive workloads. A recent study showed that 49% of nurses experience presenteeism, impacting patient care quality (Min et al., 2022). Organizational change that addresses presenteeism and prioritizes staff well-being can improve workplace culture, while personal engagement helps individuals make healthier decisions.

Self-awareness allows for change to occur. Engagement involves a new way of thinking about yourself and a new way of being. You might feel hesitant about putting time and energy into your own well-being, yet increased engagement also improves our relationships with others, helps our communities, and leads to better patient outcomes. Self-awareness is not self-consciousness. Self-consciousness makes our lives smaller, limiting our choices and flexibility. Self-awareness, on the other hand, makes our lives bigger, gives us more options, and helps us to adapt.

FINDING BALANCE

Mindfulness and Flow

Mindfulness and flow are the two sides of a coin that represents engagement. *Mindfulness* refers to intentional self-awareness and focused consciousness in a moment, and *flow* is absorption in a task when consciousness is transcended. Both are powerful tools to engage in the present.

Presence is the path to balance. Being more fully in the moment creates an experience of balance that does not involve a scorecard or counting time. Instead of focusing on making your way through the to-do list, calculating time, and wishing you could simplify, mindfulness and flow enable you to fully experience your life so that you do not feel that time is wasted, you become less vulnerable to burnout, and you achieve greater congruence and continuity in your life.

SMALL STEPS TOWARDS ENGAGEMENT

Turning off autopilot and practicing mindfulness—with intention, attention, and mindful attitudes—brings physiological changes that increase psychological flexibility and allow you to make better choices in the moment rather than relying on habit or the old default position. Practicing one mindful moment each day is a great start.

At the same time, flow allows you to turn off the inner critic, trust your skills, and become immersed in a challenging but attainable task. Flow activities boost our experience of competence and meaning in our lives and make us feel happier, more alive, and stronger. Like mindfulness practice, flow can be experienced in small moments rather than requiring a radical shift. Adjusting your skill or challenge level can bring flow to an everyday task.

Ultimately, the goal of practicing engagement is to move us out of a default position, which limits our choices. With small moments of practice, engagement can become a new default.

BALANCE BREVITIES . . . ACTION STEPS

These six tips can help guide you:

- Practice a mindful moment each day—set a timer to remind you.
- Choose one mindful attitude to practice.
- Add a challenge or goal to a task to enter flow.
- Pursue a passion.
- Increase your skill level in one activity.
- Partner with someone else in flow.

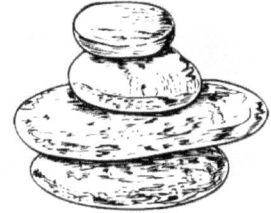

RESOURCE

MINDFULNESS

Kabat-Zinn, J. (2016). *Mindfulness for beginners: Reclaiming the present moment and your life*. Sounds True.

REFERENCES

Aust, F., Beneke, T., Peifer, C., & Wekenborg, M. (2022, March 24). The relationship between flow experience and burnout symptoms: A systematic review. *International Journal of Environmental Research and Public Health, 19*(7), 3865. https://doi.org/10.3390/ijerph19073865

Bartholomeyczik, K., Knierim, M. T., & Weinhardt, C. (2023, July 6). Fostering flow experiences at work: A framework and research agenda for developing flow interventions. *Frontiers in Psychology, 14*. https://doi.org/10.3389/fpsyg.2023.1143654

Bohlmeijer, E., Prenger, R., Taal, E., & Cuijpers, P. (2010, June). The effects of mindfulness-based stress reduction therapy on mental health of adults with a chronic medical disease: A meta-analysis. *Journal of Psychosomatic Research, 68*(6), 539–544. https://doi.org/10.1016/j.jpsychores.2009.10.005

Chander, K., Jeyaraman, M., Jeyaraman, N., & Yadav, S. (2023, Nov. 10). Presenteeism: The invisible leviathan of organizational psychology. *Cureus, 15*(11), e48620. https://doi.org/10.7759/cureus.48620

Csikszentmihalyi, M. (2008). *Flow: The psychology of optimal experience*. Harper Perennial.

Davidson, R. J., Kabat-Zinn, J., Schumacher, J., Rosenkranz, M., Muller, D., Santorelli, S. F., Urbanowski, F., Harrington, A., Bonus, K., & Sheridan, J. (2003). Alterations in brain and immune function produced by mindfulness meditation. *Psychosomatic Medicine, 65*(4), 546–570. https://doi.org/10.1097/01.PSY.0000077505.67574.E3

Flook, L., Goldberg, S. B., Pinger, L., Bonus, K., & Davidson, R. J. (2013, September). Mindfulness for teachers: A pilot study to assess effects on stress, burnout and teaching efficacy. *Mind Brain Education, 7*(3), 182–195. https://doi.org/10.1111/mbe.12026

Galante, J., Iribarren, S. J., & Pearce, P. F. (2013). Effects of mindfulness-based cognitive therapy on mental disorders: A systematic review and meta-analysis of randomised controlled trials. *Journal of Research in Nursing, 18*(2), 133–155. https://doi.org/10.1177/1744987112466087

Goodman, M. J., & Schorling, J. B. (2012). A mindfulness course decreases burnout and improves well-being among healthcare providers. *International Journal of Psychiatry in Medicine, 43*(2), 119–128. https://doi.org/10.2190/PM.43.2.b

Huskey, R. (2022, Jan. 6). *Why does experiencing 'flow' feel so good?* University of California, Davis. https://www.ucdavis.edu/curiosity/blog/research-shows-people-who-have-flow-regular-part-their-lives-are-happier-and-less-likely-focus

Jackson, S., & Eklund, R. C. (2012). Flow. In G. Tenebaum, R. C. Eklund, & A. Kamata (Eds.), *Measurement in sport and exercise psychology* (pp. 349–357). Human Kinetics.

Kabat-Zinn, J. (2013). *Full catastrophe living: Using the wisdom of your body and mind to face stress, pain, and illness* (Revised edition). Bantam.

Kabat-Zinn, J., Massion, A. O., Kristeller, J., Peterson, L. G., Fletcher, K. E., Pbert, L., Lenderking, W. R., & Santorelli, S. F. (1992, July). Effectiveness of a meditation-based stress reduction program in the treatment of anxiety disorders. *American Journal of Psychiatry, 149*(7), 936–943. https://doi.org/10.1176/ajp.149.7.936

Kral, M., & Idlout, L. (2012). It's all in the family: Well-being among Inuit in arctic Canada. In H. Selin & G. Davey (Eds.), *Happiness across cultures: Views of happiness and quality of life in non-Western cultures* (pp. 387–398). Springer Science and Business Media.

Kristeller, J. L., & Wolever, R. Q. (2011). Mindfulness-based eating awareness training for treating binge eating disorder: The conceptual foundation. *Eating Disorders, 19*(1), 49–61. https://doi.org/10.1080/10640266.2011.533605

Ledesma, D., & Kumano, H. (2009). Mindfulness-based stress reduction and cancer: A meta-analysis. *Psycho-oncology, 18*(6), 571–579. https://doi.org/10.1002/pon.1400

Maeran, R., & Cangiano, F. (2013, March). Flow experience and job characteristics: Analyzing the role of flow in job satisfaction. *TPM – Testing, Psychometrics, Methodology in Applied Psychology, 20*(1), 13–26. http://dx.doi.org/10.4473/TPM20.1.2

Min, A., Kang, M., & Park, H. (2022, October). Global prevalence of presenteeism in the nursing workforce: A meta-analysis of 28 studies from 14 countries. *Journal of Nursing Management, 30*(7), 2811–2824. https://doi.org/10.1111/jonm.13688

Nash, J. (2019, May 27). The history of meditation: Its origins & timeline. *Positive Psychology.* https://positivepsychology.com/history-of-meditation/

Shao, Y., Wu, J., Xu, W., & Zhang, C. (2024, Oct. 25). The impact of digital technology use on adolescents' subjective well-being: The serial mediating role of flow and learning engagement. *Medicine, 103*(43), e40123. https://doi.org/10.1097/MD.0000000000040123

Shapiro, S. L., Carlson, L., Astin, J., & Freedman, B. (2006, March). Mechanisms of mindfulness. *Journal of Clinical Psychology, 62*(3), 373–386. https://doi.org/10.1002/jclp.20237

Stahl, B., & Goldstein, E. (2019). *A mindfulness-based stress reduction workbook* (2nd ed.). New Harbinger Publications.

Sweeny, K., Rankin, K., Cheng, X., Hou, L., Long, F., Meng, Y., Azer, L., Zhou, R., & Zhang, W. (2020, Nov. 11). Flow in the time of COVID-19: Findings from China. *PLoS ONE, 15*(11), e0242043. https://doi.org/10.1371/journal.pone.0242043

Tabibnia, G. (2020, August). An affective neuroscience model of boosting resilience in adults. *Neuroscience & Biobehavioral Reviews, 115*, 321–350. https://doi.org/10.1016/j.neubiorev.2020.05.005

van der Linden, D., Tops, M., & Bakker, A. (2021). The neuroscience of the flow state: Involvement of the locus coeruleus norepinephrine system. *Frontiers in Psychology, 12.* https://doi.org/10.3389/fpsyg.2021.645498

Williams, K. A., Kolar, M. M., Reger, B. E., & Pearson, J. C. (2001, July). Evaluation of a wellness-based mindfulness stress reduction intervention: A controlled trial. *American Journal of Health Promotion, 15*(6), 422–432. http://dx.doi.org/10.4278/0890-1171-15.6.422

Wu, J., Xie, M., Lai, Y., Mao, Y., & Harmat, L. (2021, Nov. 15). Flow as a key predictor of subjective well-being among Chinese university students: A chain mediating model. *Frontiers in Psychology, 16*(12). https://doi.org/10.3389/fpsyg.2021.743906

II

ORGANIZATIONAL ACCOUNTABILITY & PERSONAL RESPONSIBILITY

"I have always loved my work, especially as a nurse. It's not an 'either/ or' situation because part of my life is my life's work. To me, work-life balance is more about harmony and integration of being a nurse and nurse leader as an essential ingredient of my life rather than separate spaces. I can never NOT be a nurse—and finding the blend of work as part of my life brings me energy and purpose."

–Karen Drenkard, PhD, RN, NEA-BC, FAAN
Chief Nursing Advisor, AARP Public Policy Institute

3

CREATING A SUPPORTIVE WORK ENVIRONMENT

Katie Boston-Leary, PhD, MBA, MHA, RN, NEA-BC, FADLN, FAONL

Defining Organizational Support

About the Environment

Creating a healthy work environment entails building a supportive work environment. The tenets of a healthy work environment include skilled communication, true collaboration, effective decision-making, meaningful recognition, and authentic leadership (American Association of Critical Care Nurses, 2024). These aspects of a healthy work environment foundationally require a supportive work environment that is systematically and culturally responsive to the team's needs. Teams and leaders thrive in supportive work environments, directly impacting positive outcomes.

Organizational support in the workplace is a sustained commitment and resource allocation by an employer to support the team's well-being, thereby impacting performance. This support includes policies, programs, and practices to advance mental, physical, psychological, and emotional health. Leaders foster an environment that recognizes the impact of positive and negative factors on performance, with organizations collaborating with employees and team members to mitigate issues that might otherwise lead to clinical errors, absenteeism, or reduced productivity. Effective organizational support provides employees access to resources to support their overall well-being, thus improving morale and sustaining productivity over time. There are other dividends to attain with this level of organizational support, such as improved employee engagement, reporting and reduction of clinical errors, efficiency, and innovation.

It is essential to create a supportive work environment for employees to thrive and understand how they are seen, kept safe, and supported. These efforts should be evident with transparency and accountability for all employees. This level of support should have a cascading effect from multiple levels of leadership, from the boardroom to the C-suite to the director and managerial levels. Creating a supportive work environment also requires understanding and learning from team members about what issues they need support for and how they would like to be supported.

Structures for Sustainability

How does the leadership team stay on top of the team's issues? The Motel 6 mantra "We'll leave the light on for you" is akin to the traditional open-door policies stated by leaders. An open-door policy is a start, but leaders must understand that crossing the office door threshold to surface concerns tends to be a mental hurdle for teams. Leaders must employ tactics to establish feedback and inquiry loops to understand.

How does the team escalate concerns without fear of repercussion? How do organizations consistently measure support? Deming's observation (Hunter, 2015) that you can't manage what you cannot measure is often misquoted. The more accurate context of Deming's philosophy is that while data and measurement are crucial for understanding and improving processes, not everything in an organization can be measured. Deming stressed the importance of focusing on what truly drives improvement and performance, which sometimes involves qualitative factors or human elements that cannot be easily quantified.

Regarding concerns about fear of repercussions when escalating issues, Deming would likely argue that organizations must create an environment where employees feel safe to speak up without fear of retaliation. A key principle in his work was creating a culture of trust, where individuals could openly discuss problems and suggest improvements without the threat of negative consequences. When fear prevails, it stifles innovation and growth, which ultimately harms the organization and its ability to improve.

Organizations can measure support for employees by assessing factors like trust, open communication, and the availability of resources for professional development. Tools such as employee surveys, feedback systems, and regular check-ins can help gauge whether staff feel supported. However, the true measure of support comes from the organization's actions in addressing concerns, providing guidance, and fostering an inclusive environment where all team members feel heard and valued.

FATIGUE STATS AND IMPACT ON THE WORKPLACE

Research from the National Safety Council (NSC) indicates that approximately 69% of employees report experiencing fatigue (2018). Fatigue significantly impacts individuals employed in healthcare, manufacturing, and transportation due to demanding shifts, long hours, and high-stress environments. According to the US Centers for Disease Control and Prevention (2024), 35% of US adults report not getting the recommended seven hours of sleep per night, contributing to daily fatigue that impacts workplace performance. Fatigue is known to impair cognitive function, decision-making, engagement, and overall performance. There is also evidence that fatigued workers are 70% more likely to be involved in accidents than their rested counterparts (Institute of Medicine, 2006). The economic impact of these fatigue-related errors is estimated to cost employers up to $136 billion annually (NSC, 2025), with implications for workplace injuries and harm to patients and families. Imes et al. (2023) and Trinkoff et al. (2021) addressed research from the writing group of the Expert Panel on Global Health of the American Academy of Nursing, showing that fatigued nurses are more prone to errors.

WHO OWNS FATIGUE? IT IS A TEAM SPORT.

Fatigue in the workplace is a shared responsibility between both employers and employees. Employers are responsible for creating safe, supportive work conditions that help reduce fatigue, such as manageable workloads, proper scheduling, and adequate breaks. They should also implement policies on rest, nutrition, and mental health resources to encourage a balanced work-life approach. On the other hand, employees are responsible for recognizing their own limits and taking proactive steps to manage their fatigue, including rest, seeking support when necessary, and using the tools and resources provided by their employer. Have we reached a breaking point? See the Appendix for more on recognizing a breaking point and preventive action steps.

Mutual Responsibility

Mutual responsibility in the workplace is essential for reducing fatigue-related risks by ensuring that both employers and employees actively contribute to creating a healthy, balanced environment. Employers should prioritize well-being through reasonable workloads, breaks, and support systems. At the same time, employees must engage in self-love, self-care, system-care, and system-engagement (see Figure 3.1), and should communicate when feeling overwhelmed, fostering a culture of collaboration and proactive risk management.

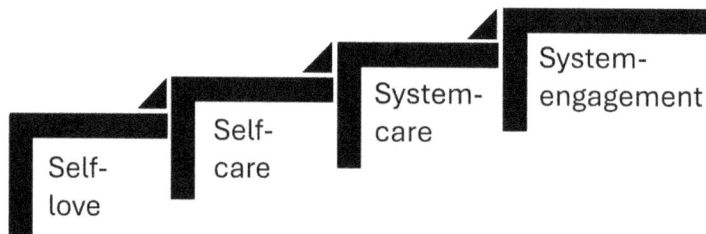

FIGURE 3.1 The need to honor self.

Individual Level

As CEOs of our overall health and well-being, we must use discernment in what activities we engage in and how much—particularly the ones that do not benefit us, those that we care for, and those that we love. As clinicians, we must discard our rescuer identities, where we sacrifice so much of our care in exchange for the care of others. To care for ourselves, we must love ourselves as a first step. In this case, it is not only about knowing that you love yourself and are meeting your basic needs but also about what you do beyond that: care for yourself and choose to stop engaging in activities that are harmful to you physically and psychologically. The love that truly manifests at the individual level resists the temptation and pressures to place your care on the back burner for a sustained time and choose yourself.

System Level

Where individuals or teams go, the system goes. Systems should own the overall care and well-being of the individuals and teams within the system like never before. When individuals are thriving and feel cared for, people within the system experience bouts of joy, and the system is cared for, translating into patients and families feeling cared for. Joy for the people who work within systems happens when they engage in meaningful, value-added, and less burdensome work. This is important to note because we have unintentionally and systematically created systems where clinicians spend less and less time with patients. Strategic plans should consistently advance efforts to address all facets of their employees' well-being and measure success from a process perspective—and, most importantly, an outcomes perspective. Innovation and culling of innovative ideas co-created with the employees within the system are critical for the sustainment of the teams within. This effort goes beyond the traditional employee assistance programs, quiet rooms, and pedometer competitions. Gallup's Well-being at Work (Clifton & Harter, 2024) framework addresses the need to structurally support social, community, financial, physical, and career teams. Lastly, organization leaders should resist cutting programs when financial pressures arise. These investments are needed to care for the team systematically and reflect that the organization cares! Caring for teams in innovative ways could be a market differentiator to secure top talent from a recruitment and retention perspective, particularly in a highly competitive market.

THE SYSTEM AND IMPACT OF FATIGUE ON PERFORMANCE

The broader system within which an organization operates, including industry standards, regulations, and cultural expectations, plays a significant role in shaping workplace fatigue. Regulatory bodies may set mandatory rest periods and work-hour limitations or provide guidelines to help prevent employee fatigue in specific high-stakes industries like healthcare, transportation, or manufacturing. Fatigue significantly affects performance by impairing cognitive and physical functions, leading to slower reaction times, decreased concentration, and higher error rates. When organizational support is lacking, employees are more vulnerable to fatigue's negative impacts, which can, in turn, jeopardize productivity, safety, and overall job satisfaction.

IMPACT OF WORKLOAD ON FATIGUE

If systems can meaningfully address the workload issues in healthcare, it will be a game changer. Workload issues have plagued healthcare for too long without much progress, and that is with the supposed additive benefits of technology. We must ask ourselves why this continues to be the case. Healthcare's top talents are leaving acute care settings for ambulatory settings and healthcare overall for areas and industries that are less workload-intense and more amenable to providing balance and harmony for work and life. Based on feedback from clinicians, we know that work within healthcare tends to be physically, emotionally, mentally, and cognitively taxing on a sustained basis, with the only potential reprieve to occur during brief moments of rest. There should be a relentless pursuit and drive to unearth new strategies to reduce workload.

FINDING ☙ BALANCE

Workload

Merriam-Webster (n.d.) defines workload as:

"The amount of work or of working time expected or assigned and the amount of work performed or capable of being performed (as by a mechanical device) usually within a specific period."

Keywords to focus on in this definition are *assigned, amount,* and *capable.*

Assigned: How much should a nurse be responsible for delivering high-quality care? Who determines the need to reassess and amend assignments when they become overwhelming? What technologies are available to measure the real-time impact of workload and performance?

Amount: What are the determinants of how nurses are assigned and when to call for support? What is baked in the system for workload, and were nurses caring for patients involved in building these formulas?

Capable: How do we understand the impact of demand versus capacity on nurses? Are we measuring capability solely based on competence and training? What other measures exist to understand capacity and capability in real time?

Understanding how to manage workload in terms of assignment, the amount of work distributed, and the capability and capacity of nurses and healthcare professionals is the innovation opportunity that must be realized for a better future. A true team approach and intentional and equity-minded collaboration are the keys to unlocking our greatest potential where we can all flourish while achieving relative balance and harmony in our personal and professional lives.

TEAMWORK AND COLLABORATION

Teamwork and collaboration are essential elements of a productive and positive workplace. When team members work well together, they can leverage diverse skills, perspectives, and strengths, which breeds a positive work environment where innovation and joy happen. The premise here is not to suggest that teamwork has not occurred in healthcare or nursing; we are stating that we can engage with each other differently. I love this quote:

"Leadership in the fourth industrial revolution will be defined by the ability to rapidly align and engage empowered, networked teams with a clarity of purpose and a fierce resolve to win."

–Brian Bacon
Chair and founder of Oxford Leadership

Let's unpack Bacon's statement to illustrate its applicability to nursing and healthcare.

Rapid alignment occurs when leaders and the team understand their shared purpose. This sets up a clear vision that every team member can sink their teeth into. Everyone on the team strongly desires to achieve the vision, and there is mutual agreement on what it takes to get there:

- Empowered and networked teams understand their collective power and the strength of their interdependence. They do not fear leveraging that power to own the strategy, accountability, and results.

- *Clarity of purpose* is all team members being clear-eyed about their whys. It is understanding that every team member has the power to be anywhere else but chooses on their own volition to be a part of this charge, this opportunity, this movement that could impact the lives of many others. With clarity of purpose comes pride in understanding and articulating why we do what we do.

- *Fierce resolve to win* is interesting here, particularly in healthcare, because we don't usually see our day-to-day work as winning. It is mainly viewed (understandably) as a grind to get things done; the goal is to get through the day. There is a significant opportunity for a reset here. What should *win* mean in healthcare? Every leader should set an expectation or goal of what winning looks like every day for the team to have something to build toward by the end of the day. Will everyone get quality breaks? Will all expected discharges be completed by a specific time? Is it possible for every team member to be safe from injury? Small and recognized wins inch toward the larger vision every minute, every hour, and every day. We do not look for and celebrate wins in healthcare as standard work. This helps address perceptions of daily defeat and compassion fatigue that healthcare professionals face. How can leaders help set the tone for what winning looks like daily?

A collaborative work environment encourages open communication, trust, and mutual support, fostering unity and shared purpose. Organizations prioritizing teamwork improve individual performance and create an environment where employees feel valued and supported, leading to higher job satisfaction and employee retention.

"In today's dynamic and ever-changing healthcare landscape, resources are constantly being depleted, leading to exhaustion of our nursing staff. To survive these challenges, nurses must prioritize well-being, not just for themselves but for their team as well. Well-being strategies that focus on the team as a unit help lighten the workload, strengthen the team's foundation, and empower nurses to thrive together."

–Frankie Hamilton, MBA, MSN, RN, NEA-BC, FACHE
Vice President of Nursing Operations, Maimonides Medical Center

---

PROMOTING A CULTURE OF TEAMWORK AND COLLABORATION

According to an article in *Harvard Business Review* (Burkus, 2023) on building trust in teams, teamwork is essential for providing care and is therefore prominent in healthcare organizations. However:

- A lack of teamwork is often identified as a primary point of vulnerability for quality and safety of care.

- Research found that high-performing teams are exceedingly rare; only 8.7% of respondents gave their teams high scores (Burkus, 2023).

Creating a culture emphasizing teamwork and collaboration requires intentional effort and structured strategies. It is also essential to recognize that everyone contributes certain intangibles differently. The intangibles are not covered in job descriptions or role clarity formalities but in what people are known for within the team. A standard operating procedure on the individual level that informs teams provides clarity on how people interact, how they can be engaged, and what they are best able to do within the team.

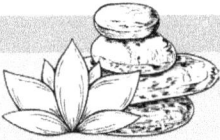

DESIGNING HARMONY EXERCISE 3.1

Manual of Me

I am at my best when _____.

I am at my worst when _____.

You can count on me to _____.

What I need from you is _____.

Source: Burkus, 2023

43

Organizations can encourage collaboration by implementing team-building activities, providing cross-functional projects, and creating open, flexible office spaces that facilitate interaction. Encouraging transparent communication, where employees feel comfortable sharing ideas and asking questions, also strengthens collaboration. By providing tools and platforms for seamless communication, such as project management software and video conferencing tools, employers can help teams collaborate effectively, even when working remotely.

LEADERSHIP'S ROLE IN FOSTERING COLLABORATION

Leaders play a critical role in cultivating a collaborative work environment. Influential leaders model teamwork by being approachable, showing empathy, and encouraging open dialogue among team members. Leaders also model collaboration by how they appear to their teams working with other leaders and departments within the organization. If you are consistently at odds with other department leaders and do not find ways to work through those issues in good faith, that will show up within the teams of those leaders. It is always good to remember that you are constantly on stage as a leader and that we work within networks—that is, people talk.

Leaders should also recognize and reward collaborative efforts, reinforcing the importance of teamwork in the organization. Treat small wins as important as big wins. It also helps to create a lesson learned so that as much as the team wants to win, there is no losing when goals are not met – there is learning (see Figure 3.2). This powerful visual metaphor highlights the mindset shift necessary for success: Every outcome, whether expected or not, is an opportunity for growth. By embracing learning as a natural part of the journey, individuals can reframe setbacks as stepping stones to future success, ensuring that every goal pursued contributes to continuous improvement and development. Additionally, leaders can facilitate collaboration by setting clear goals, aligning team efforts with organizational objectives, and providing the necessary resources for team members to work effectively. Leaders can motivate employees to contribute their best to the team by promoting inclusivity and a sense of belonging.

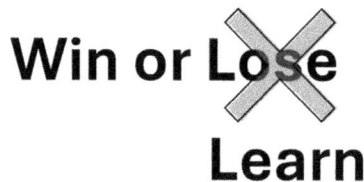

Win or Lose

Learn

FIGURE 3.2 From win or lose to win or learn.

ADDRESSING STRESS IN TEAM ENVIRONMENTS

Collaboration can sometimes introduce stress, especially when team members face tight deadlines, unclear roles, or conflicting ideas. While collaboration can be beneficial, if not managed carefully, it may also lead to misunderstandings or over-dependence, where certain team members feel pressured to take on more responsibility. Organizations should establish clear communication channels to mitigate stress, define roles, and set realistic expectations. Leaders can help manage team stress by addressing issues promptly, promoting a culture of respect, and offering support when conflicts arise. Encouraging breaks and promoting work-life balance are also vital in reducing stress.

BENEFITS OF A COLLABORATIVE AND SUPPORTIVE WORK ENVIRONMENT

A workplace that values teamwork and collaboration fosters a supportive environment where employees feel connected to their colleagues and the organization—creating the foundation for a psychologically safe space where everyone feels heard, respected, and empowered to contribute. Such an environment can lead to greater resilience, as team members support one another during challenging times. Furthermore, the collective intelligence of a well-coordinated team often results in improved problem-solving and innovation, ultimately enhancing the organization's ability to adapt and grow. By emphasizing teamwork, organizations benefit from a productive, motivated, and engaged workforce, setting the stage for sustained success.

BALANCE BREVITIES . . . ACTION STEPS

Here are four action steps for creating a supportive work environment:

1. Implement clear communication and feedback channels.
2. Prioritize well-being through organizational policies.
3. Empower and align teams with a shared purpose.
4. Invest in leadership development and role-modeling, and advocate for resources to maintain a positive and productive environment.

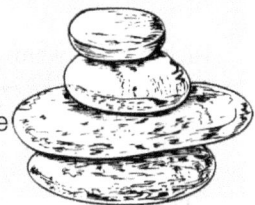

REFERENCES

American Association of Critical Care Nurses. (2024, April). *Healthy work environments national collaborative.* https://www.aacn.org/nursing-excellence/healthy-work-environments/hwe-national-collaborative

Burkus, D. (2023, Aug. 29). What makes some teams high performing? *Harvard Business Review.* https://hbr.org/2023/08/what-makes-some-teams-high-performing

Clifton, J., & Harter, J. (2024). *Wellbeing at work: How to build resilient and thriving teams.* Gallup.

Hunter, J. (2015, Aug. 13). *Myth: If you can't measure it, you can't manage it.* The Deming Institute. https://deming.org/myth-if-you-cant-measure-it-you-cant-manage-it/

Imes, C. C., Tucker, S. J., Trinkoff, A. M., Chasens, E. R., Weinstein, S. M., Dunbar-Jacob, J., Patrician, P. A., Redeker, N. S., & Baldwin, C. M. (2023). Wake-up call: Night shifts adversely affect nurse health and retention, patient and public safety, and costs. *Nursing Administration Quarterly, 47*(4), E38–E53. https://doi.org/10.1097/NAQ.0000000000000595

Institute of Medicine. (2006). *Sleep disorders and sleep deprivation: An unmet public health problem.* National Academies Press. https://www.ncbi.nlm.nih.gov/books/NBK19958/

Merriam-Webster. (n.d.). Workload. In *Merriam-Webster.com dictionary.* https://www.merriam-webster.com/dictionary/workload

National Safety Council. (2018, Oct. 1). *69% of employees, many of them in safety-critical jobs, are tired at work.* https://www.nsc.org/in-the-newsroom/69-percent-of-employees-many-in-safety-critical-jobs-are-tired-at-work-says-nsc-report?srsltid=AfmBOooe7HF4z1xByGFpHmSTBKguH-OrIEonRvSE4ct4WHlnB5v_RXX5

National Safety Council. (2025). *Cost of fatigue in the workplace.* https://www.nsc.org/workplace/safety-topics/fatigue/cost-of-fatigue-at-work?srsltid=AfmBOorUKxnmXAoUusoQSspNJj6w98TADmD9uYMrfqjt5L7r2TudTG4V

Trinkoff, A. M., Baldwin, C. M., Chasens, E. R., Dunbar-Jacob, J., Geiger-Brown, J., Imes, C. C., Landis, C. A., Patrician, P. A., Redeker, N. S., Rogers, A. E., Scott, L. D., Todero, C. M., Tucker, S. J., Weinstein, S. M., Fatigue Subgroup of the Health Behavior Expert Panel, & American Academy of Nursing. (2021). Nurses are more exhausted than ever: What should we do about it? *American Journal of Nursing, 121*(12), 18–28. https://doi.org/10.1097/01.NAJ.0000802688.16426.8d

US Centers for Disease Control and Prevention. (2024, June 3). : *Sleep.* https://www.cdc.gov/cdi/indicator-definitions/sleep.html

4

STRATEGIES FOR WORK/LIFE HARMONY

Katie Boston-Leary, PhD, MBA, MHA, RN, NEA-BC, FADLN, FAONL

THE WORK/LIFE BALANCE CONUNDRUM: IS BALANCING WORK AND LIFE A FALLACY?

Since the COVID-19 pandemic, many well-being concepts, including work-life balance, have been challenged. Commonly, *work-life balance* is defined as giving equal time to personal and professional activities. Sirgy (2023) suggests balancing job time with family and leisure, implying no joy in work. In Shiftbase, the author cites prioritizing responsibilities to ensure well-being, suggesting individuals are solely responsible for achieving balance (Bonifacio, 2024). However, this raises the question: Is "balance" the right goal, and can it be achieved?

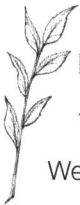

HARMONY REFLECTION

Work-Life vs. Life-Work

We have seen shifts in the concept of work-life balance:

- **Life-work balance:** Prioritizes life over work.
- **Work-life integration:** Blends both worlds for compromise.
- **Work-life harmony:** Incorporates work into life to promote happiness both at home and work.

Which concept should we adopt? It's unclear as ideas continue to evolve. Regardless of the definition, consider the following:

- How we define and use concepts in our lives is personal.
- There is no right or wrong.
- We should permit ourselves to fail sometimes.
- Our priorities change over time.
- We are human "beings," after all.
- Work-life balance is a continuum.

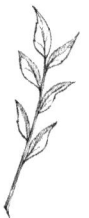

This is personal.

Sometimes, we get so close to a goal or achievement that we must briefly reprioritize work over life, like during the final school semesters. Similarly, in personal situations, we might prioritize family when a loved one needs us, checking entirely out of work for a period. The challenge is knowing how long is too long and how to monitor the trend to ensure balance, integration, or harmony.

Options, not absolutes.

How do we know if we're managing life and work correctly? We often regret past actions and wish for a redo with the knowledge we have now. However, our lives are unique, and comparing ourselves to others isn't fair. Everyone navigates life differently.

Permission to fail and falter.

There's no road map for achieving harmony. Mistakes, including repeated ones, are part of the journey. Not achieving or constantly striving to achieve balance or harmony doesn't mean we've failed. Each new day offers a fresh start, and we must allow ourselves grace when we fall short, learning and growing from the experience to be better each day.

Shifting priorities.

Navigating life and its challenges requires flexibility and adaptability. We need to adjust accordingly, stay nimble, and allow ourselves the grace to shift priorities when needed. Shifting our priorities does not necessarily mean we are indecisive, frivolous, or undisciplined. We are human, after all.

Being human means recognizing our fragilities and imperfections. We make mistakes, learn, and grow. In the work-life continuum, we must address our needs, remembering Maslow's Hierarchy of Needs (King, 2024). Physiological needs always come first. Meeting your physiological needs first is fundamental and foremost. In the busyness of life, we often forget this natural order and must remind ourselves to prioritize these fundamental needs. It is a continuum.

Managing work and life is an ongoing process that varies. The key is recognizing where we are and adjusting to improve continually. Each day is a new opportunity to be better than before.

Life-work harmony is an evolving process that integrates personal and professional responsibilities seamlessly, allowing both to thrive without compromise. Unlike rigid "balance," harmony emphasizes fluidity, alignment, and adaptability to life's changing priorities. It involves setting boundaries, prioritizing values, and ensuring work complements life. Flexible schedules, meaningful goals, and quality time with loved ones foster well-being and reduce stress. Employers play a key role by supporting holistic wellness, while individuals must practice self-awareness and time management. At its core, life-work harmony ensures work enhances life, creating a dynamic, productive, and fulfilling experience that adapts to every stage of life. See Chapters 1, 2, and 7.

Healthy Nurse, Healthy Nation

The American Nurses Association's (ANA) Healthy Nurse, Healthy Nation (HNHN) initiative is a free program available to nurses and others interested in becoming a part of a community focused on overall well-being. HNHN was formed in 2017 after ANA leaders noted nurses' alarmingly poor well-being statistics compared to other professionals. HNHN offers a heat map survey to assess domains of well-being, such as quality of life, sleep, nutrition, physical activity, mental health, and safety. Nurses can participate as individuals or through organizations. The motto of HNHN is "Healing the nation, one nurse at a time."

What Is a Healthy Nurse?

Engaging with HNHN pulls you into a community of nurses and other professionals to learn and share ideas on striving for health and well-being. HNHN just revisited and revised its definition of a healthy nurse.

Old: "A healthy nurse actively focuses on creating and maintaining a balance and synergy of physical, intellectual, emotional, social, spiritual, financial, personal, and professional well-being. A healthy nurse lives life to the fullest capacity, across the wellness/illness continuum, as they become stronger role models, advocates, and educators, personally, for their families, communities, work environments, and patients."

New: "A healthy nurse prioritizes striving toward positive physical, mental, social, environmental, and professional well-being."

Prioritizing and Striving

The new healthy nurse definition includes two keywords for nurses to take better care of themselves—prioritizing and striving. The importance of these words is critical when so much is required of nurses with limited capacity to expand to accommodate more. That overwhelming demand compared to capacity leads to stress and then, if unmanaged, burnout, depression, and suicide ideation (see Chapter 7). Intentional action is required in an atmosphere that creates so much whiplash and limited recovery ability. *Prioritizing* requires nurses to put themselves first and certain actions first to resist not doing so and sacrifice self-care for other care. *Striving* entails acknowledging what nurses are up against. Given the environment and how it can easily deter nurses from doing what is needed to take better care of themselves, nurses must fight and push against the current to force care for themselves structurally, meaningfully, and consistently.

What Does HNHN Offer Individuals to Manage the Continuum?

HNHN offers an online platform, emails, texts, and social media for nurses and student nurses to connect with and support each other, engage in friendly competition, expand their wellness knowledge and expertise, and assess and track their health and wellness progress. There is a commitment wall, discussion boards, health and wellness blogs, nurse and organizational spotlight stories, comprehensive health surveys with immediate results, monthly wellness challenges, giveaways, coffee chats, and special events. See Figure 4.1

What Does HNHN Offer Partner Organizations?

As a free nurse wellness program for your organization, HNHN offers partner organizations a monthly newsletter and recognition opportunities via blogs and spotlights on the website and social media platforms if they join at certain partner levels (all levels are free!). Organizations can receive de-identified, aggregated data reports after 25 or more participants take the health survey and affiliate with their organization. Learn more at hnhn.org.

FINDING ✿ BALANCE

Getting Started With HNHN

You can participate in various ways:

- Join the online platform at hnhn.org
- Receive monthly text challenge tips by texting healthynurse to 52886
- Request to join the Facebook group (Healthy Nurse, Healthy Nation)

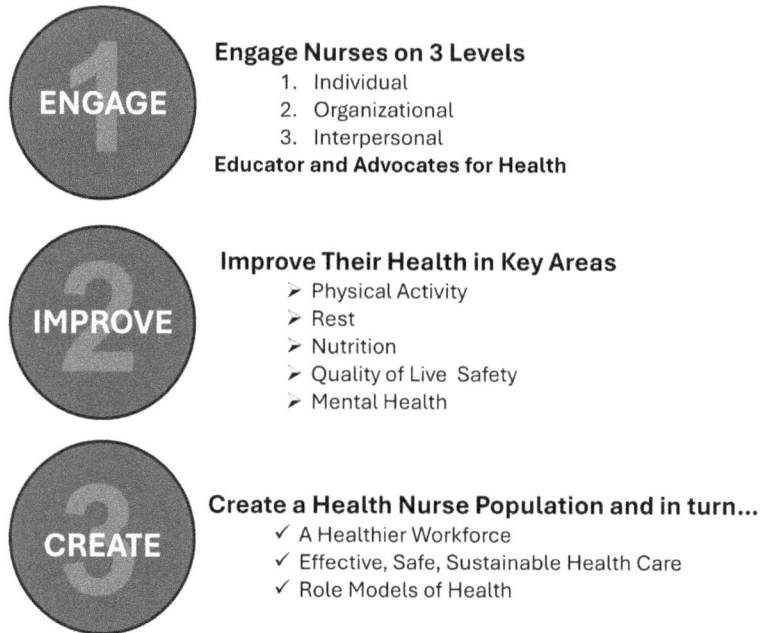

Engage Nurses on 3 Levels
1. Individual
2. Organizational
3. Interpersonal
Educator and Advocates for Health

Improve Their Health in Key Areas
➤ Physical Activity
➤ Rest
➤ Nutrition
➤ Quality of Live Safety
➤ Mental Health

Create a Health Nurse Population and in turn...
✓ A Healthier Workforce
✓ Effective, Safe, Sustainable Health Care
✓ Role Models of Health

FIGURE 4.1   Healthy Nurse, Healthy Nation Implementation Model.

"Healthcare is getting more complex, and nurses must prioritize their own physical, intellectual, personal, and professional well-being. Achieving this will enable nurses to handle the demands of the profession."

–Michelle A. Chester, DNP, MSN, BSN, RN, FNP-BC
Northwell Health

The HNHN Care Plan

HNHN offers a well-being framework modeled on a nursing care plan (see Figure 4.2). Nurses assess well-being via the Healthy Nurse Survey, diagnose needs, and plan interventions. Strategies are implemented alongside educational resources explaining their importance. Finally, a post-intervention survey evaluates the impact on healthy behaviors, fostering continuous improvement in nurse well-being.

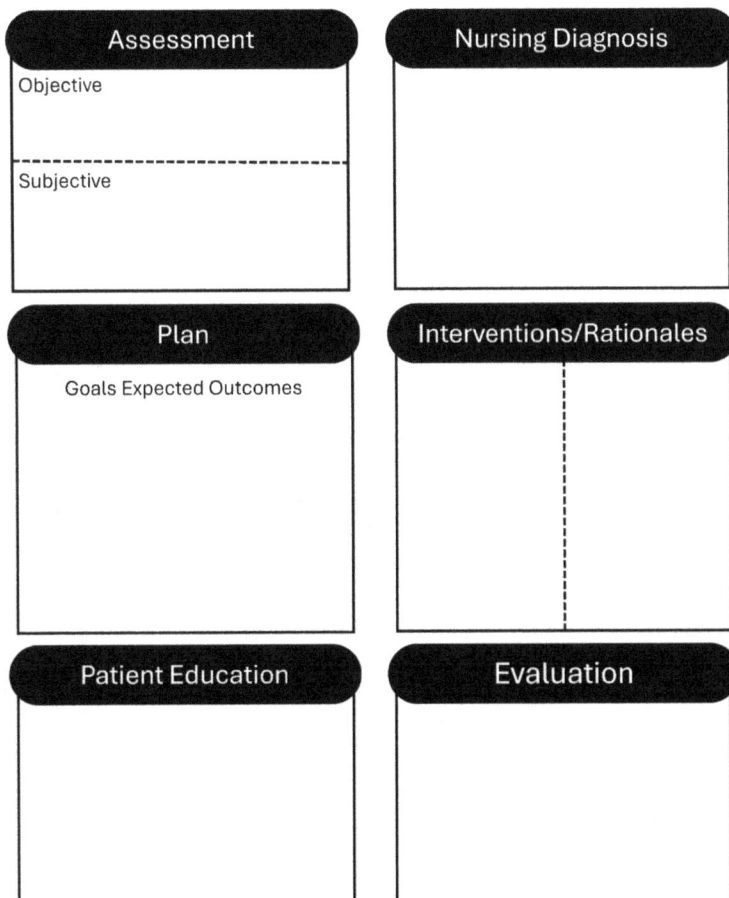

FIGURE 4.2   Nursing care plan.

AMERICAN ASSOCIATION OF COLLEGES OF NURSING (AACN) *ESSENTIALS*

The new AACN (2021) guide emphasizes diversity, equity, and inclusion and urges activism against social injustice and structural racism. Through this broad perspective, nurses approach their profession to achieve the best possible patient outcomes. The document outlines 10 core domains and key competence areas, providing a comprehensive framework for nursing practice:

1. Knowledge for Nursing Practice

2. Person-Centered Care

3. Population Health

4. Scholarship for Nursing Discipline

5. Quality and Safety

6. Interprofessional Partnerships

7. Systems-Based Practice

8. Informatics and Healthcare Technologies

9. Professionalism

10. Personal, Professional, and Leadership Development

ANA also offers resources on how to address inequities within the profession, in nursing practice and work settings. The National Commission to Address Racism in Nursing has compiled an Actionable Allyship Self-Assessment Tool for nurses to better advocate for themselves, each other, and patients within their care (ANA, 2021). Access it here:

https://www.nursingworld.org/globalassets/practiceandpolicy/workforce/
commission-to-address-racism/ana-allyship-self-assesment-form.pdf

Actionable allyship (see the graphic below) is defined as the intentional use of interventions, advocacy, and support to:

- Eliminate harmful actions and words
- Create space for and strengthen voices that may not typically be heard, recognized, or welcome

To be an ally you must act.

To act you must know.

To know you must learn.

And to learn you must listen.

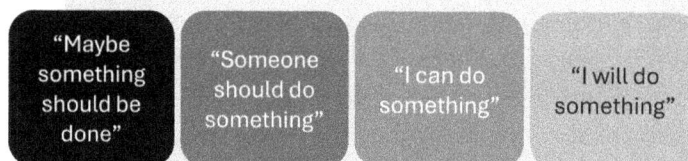

The HNHN initiative aligns with the AACN *Essentials* by promoting holistic health and well-being among nurses, which is integral to achieving the competencies outlined in the AACN *Essentials*. Here's how the HNHN initiative supports the *Essentials*:

- Patient-Centered Care

- Teamwork and Collaboration

- Evidence-Based Practice

- Quality Improvement

- Safety

- Informatics

See the Appendix for more details.

Harmony in the Balance

Harmony in balance is about recognizing that achieving optimal well-being is a journey, not a destination. It's about understanding and accepting the effort required to maintain good health and well-being. For nurses, balance and harmony are vital in enhancing their physical, emotional, mental, and spiritual health while navigating the demands of their profession. Gallup's well-being-at-work framework (Clifton & Harter, 2021) highlights the importance of social, community, career, physical, and financial well-being in this process. Achieving harmony means integrating these aspects of life, ensuring meaningful connections, career satisfaction, physical activity, and economic stability.

Balance, however, involves managing life's demands without neglecting self-care. It requires setting boundaries, prioritizing responsibilities, and ensuring time for rest and rejuvenation. Balance fosters personal growth and prevents burnout, helping to allocate energy wisely across work, relationships, and leisure. Individuals create a foundation for long-term happiness and success by striving for balance and harmony.

Synchronicity represents the sweet spot where life and work flow seamlessly. It results from prioritizing and striving toward harmony, leading to thriving in both realms. Synchronicity is dynamic, not static, and aligns one's values, priorities, and actions across all areas of life. It enhances well-being, creativity, and fulfillment, reducing stress while fostering growth. When work and life align synchronously, energy flows between both domains, contributing to a unified, fulfilling existence. This space of harmony serves as a touchstone, helping us navigate challenges when they arise (see Chapter 2). Figure 4.3 shows how synchronicity and balance emphasize dynamic adaptability over perfection.

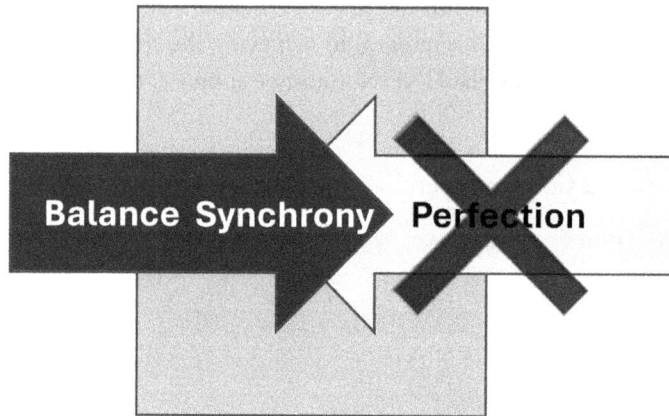

FIGURE 4.3 Synchronicity.

"Synchronicity is an ever-present reality for those who
have eyes to see."

–Carl Jung, psychologist

PERSONAL HEALTH AND WELLNESS

Well-being is personal in terms of uniqueness, opportunities, and actions. Personal health and wellness encompass nurses' physical, emotional, and mental well-being. These factors are deeply interrelated, influencing how we feel and perform daily activities. The old saying that where the mind goes, the body goes rings true here. Achieving harmony in health requires attention to lifestyle choices and preferences, including nutrition, exercise, sleep, and mental health practices. It also involves self-awareness and adaptability, recognizing the unique needs of one's body and mind. Personal wellness is not just about preventing illness but advancing wellness—thriving to support long-term vitality and happiness.

"As you race through your job, whether in healthcare or not, remember to take those critical moments to pull the car over and check the gas. Story is the fuel you need and doesn't cost you anything. No matter what lies ahead, you can face it with passion, purpose, and possibility as long as you know how to frame it. Story reaches where medicine can't."

–Kelly Swanson, CSP, CPAE, extraordinary storyteller

MANAGING FATIGUE

Fatigue can impact productivity, mood, and well-being. To manage it, identify root causes like poor sleep, stress, or medical conditions. Prioritize restorative sleep, a balanced diet, hydration, and regular exercise. Use mindfulness, meditation, and relaxation to manage stress, and practice time management and realistic goal-setting to maintain energy.

GUT CHECK: HOW DO I FEEL?

Regularly checking in with oneself to ask "How do I feel?" is a powerful practice for enhancing personal health. This introspection involves assessing physical sensations, emotional states, and mental clarity. As we engage and interact with people throughout the day, pausing and checking in is crucial. This is the "being" part of our humanity. We tend to skip over understanding our feelings before reacting to things happening around us. It should be part of how we act, like crossing the street. Good questions to ask yourself to check in are:

- Am I in a good mental space?

- What am I reacting to?

- Does it warrant a reaction in the moment?

- Can it wait?

- Can I make the situation better, or will I make it worse?

Acknowledging feelings without judgment or fear creates space for addressing unmet needs or imbalances. For example, irritability or sadness may indicate stress or a need for connection, while physical discomfort may signal the need for rest or medical attention. Expressing emotions constructively promotes resilience and self-compassion. The emotion wheel helps identify and understand emotions, starting with broad categories and narrowing down to specific feelings. There is a saying that "if you name it, you can tame it!" It enhances emotional awareness, vocabulary, and regulation, helping you process your emotions or connect with others (Willcox, 1982).

The emotion wheel, or feelings wheel, is a visual tool that maps out a wide range of emotions in a circular layout (see Figure 4.4). It starts with broad categories of feelings and then breaks them into more specific, nuanced emotions.

Use it to identify and understand your emotions more clearly. By showing various feelings, the emotion wheel makes pinpointing your feelings easier. It's especially helpful for building a richer emotional vocabulary improving emotional awareness, intelligence, and regulation. Whether you're trying to process your emotions or connect with someone else's, the emotion wheel can guide you to a deeper understanding of how emotions work (Willcox, 1982).

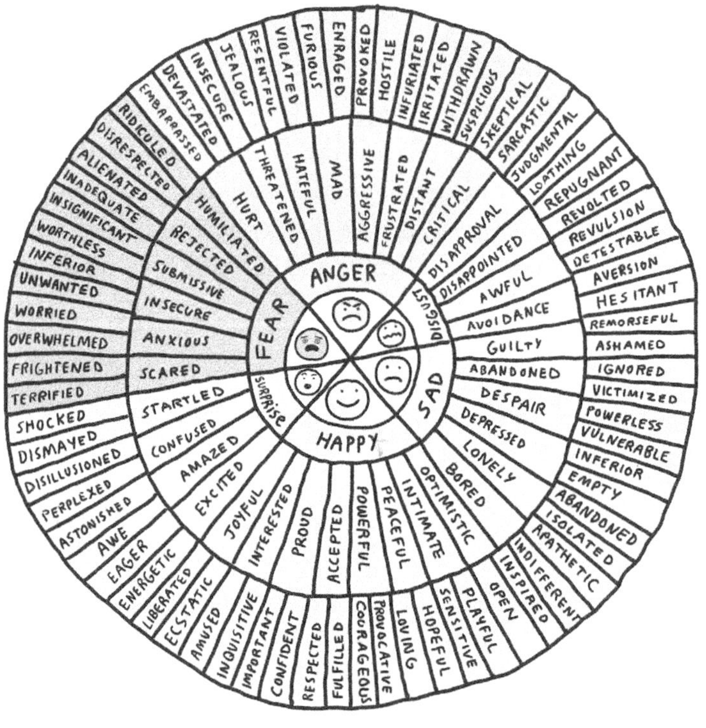

FIGURE 4.4   Wheel of emotions
(Willcox, 1982; modified by Hallie Bateman, 2022 @hallithbates Instagram).

HEEDING TO ONE'S BODY

Listening to one's body is a fundamental aspect of wellness, requiring attention to subtle cues like hunger, fatigue, or pain. This practice aligns with Maslow's body assessment. For instance, feeling thirsty prompts hydration, while persistent fatigue requires rest or medical evaluation. By tuning into these signals, individuals can make informed decisions about diet, exercise, and health, avoiding harm to themselves and those around them. Ignoring these signals can lead to physical and emotional strain. This process fosters a deeper connection with oneself, promoting long-term well-being. By caring for ourselves, we place ourselves in a better position to serve and support others, recognizing that self-love and self-care are integral to overall health.

SELF-REGULATION

Self-regulation is the ability to manage emotions, thoughts, and behaviors in alignment with long-term goals and values. Acting as the CEO of our feelings promotes thoughtful actions and constructive interactions, which are essential for emotional balance, healthy relationships, and personal success. Self-regulation leads to fewer regrets by fostering measured responses instead of impulsive reactions, bringing individuals closer to Maslow's self-actualization.

Developing self-regulation requires awareness and consistent practice. Mindfulness and deep breathing help maintain calm under pressure, while clear goals and manageable steps prevent overwhelm. Regular self-reflection helps evaluate actions, identify triggers, and develop better strategies for future challenges. Over time, these habits strengthen resilience and self-control, reducing emotional reactions and enhancing logical decision-making through the brain's frontal lobes. See Chapter 2.

Robust self-regulation improves personal and professional life by reducing stress, fostering empathy, and enhancing communication. It boosts productivity in high-pressure environments and empowers individuals to align their actions with core values, promoting a balanced and fulfilling life. Self-regulation becomes a cornerstone of well-being by managing stress and preventing emotional overwhelm, paving the way for meaningful success and stronger relationships.

Self-Regulating

According to sources (Cuncic, 2023; Hampson et al., 2016; Yeow & Martin, 2013), self-regulators, those who are adept at self-regulating, can:

- Act in accordance with their values
- Calm themselves when upset
- Cheer themselves when feeling down
- Maintain open communication
- Persist through difficult times
- Put forth their best effort
- Remain flexible and adapt to situations
- See the good in others
- Stay clear about their intentions
- Take control of situations when necessary
- View challenges as opportunities

The Two Wolves: A Native American Tale

An old Cherokee was teaching his grandchildren about life. He said, "A battle is raging inside me . . . it is a terrible fight between two wolves. One wolf represents fear, anger, envy, sorrow, regret, greed, arrogance, self-pity, guilt, resentment, inferiority, lies, false pride, superiority, and ego. The other stands for joy, peace, love, hope, sharing, serenity, humility, kindness, benevolence, friendship, empathy, generosity, truth, compassion, and faith."

The old man looked at the children with a firm stare. "This same fight is going on inside you, and inside every other person too."

The children thought about it for a minute, and then one child asked his grandfather, "Which wolf will win?"

The old Cherokee replied, "The one you feed."

Source: College of Education at the University of Texas at Austin, 2025

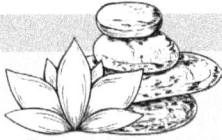

Feeding the Good Wolf: Keys to Self-Regulation

1. Manage your Maslow's basic needs such as sleep, technological rest, nutrition, breathing, etc.

2. Connect with others to avoid social isolation.

3. Find your outlet and what feeds your spirit.

4. Again, breathe!

5. Journal—write it down!

6. Pause and check your sternum—this is the heaviness in your chest that you feel when you feel threatened, upset, or mistreated.

7. Evaluate your actions.

CULTIVATING A WELLNESS ROUTINE

A holistic approach to health and wellness blends proactive habits with self-awareness. Establishing a daily routine that includes enough sleep, nutritious meals, regular exercise, and time for mental relaxation forms a strong foundation for well-being. Practicing mindfulness and gratitude promotes a positive outlook, while engaging in hobbies or social interactions enriches life. Ultimately, health and wellness are about harmonizing the body, mind, and spirit, empowering individuals to live vibrant, fulfilling lives (American Holistic Health Association, n.d.; Bowen College, n.d.; Wisner, 2024).

GRIT: THE POWER OF PERSEVERANCE

Grit is the unwavering strength of character that empowers individuals to persist through challenges, setbacks, and adversity. It combines passion and sustained effort, allowing people to achieve long-term goals. Grit goes beyond talent or intelligence; it reflects resilience, perseverance, and a commitment to overcoming obstacles. Those who cultivate grit face challenges with determination, seeing failure as a learning opportunity. This mindset fosters a deep sense of purpose, motivating individuals to progress despite difficulties.

In her book *Grit: The Power of Passion and Perseverance* (2016), Angela Duckworth highlights key principles for developing grit:

- **Passion:** Grit involves maintaining consistent interest in a goal over time. Passion is about persistence, not intensity, staying committed even when enthusiasm wanes.

- **Perseverance:** Grit requires long-term effort, especially through setbacks. Success often comes from steady progress, not quick victories.

Duckworth (2016) identifies four essential components of grit:

1. **Interest:** Genuine enjoyment and curiosity about what you do.

2. **Practice:** Deliberate practice to continually improve your skills.

3. **Purpose:** Belief that your work contributes to something greater than yourself.

4. **Hope:** The belief that you can overcome adversity and keep pushing forward.

A "gritty culture" can also inspire perseverance, as surrounding yourself with like-minded, persistent individuals fosters these qualities in yourself. Cultivating grit involves showing up consistently in personal and professional endeavors. By embracing endurance, tenacity, and emotional intelligence, individuals navigate life's complexities with confidence and resilience. Grit drives personal success, motivates others to pursue their goals, and fosters a team-growth mindset.

ENDURANCE

Endurance is a critical aspect of grit, allowing individuals to persist through physical or mental challenges over time. It involves withstanding fatigue, stress, and discomfort while staying focused on long-term goals. Building endurance requires consistent effort, whether training for a marathon or meeting demanding deadlines. The key to endurance is pacing oneself, prioritizing self-care, and maintaining a long-term perspective.

TENACITY

Tenacity reflects the determination to push forward despite obstacles. Fueled by belief in one's abilities, tenacious individuals adapt to setbacks, using creativity and problem-solving skills to overcome challenges.

RECOVERY AND RESTORATION

Recovery is essential for sustained success. While persistence is vital, rest and rejuvenation are necessary to prevent burnout. Practices like mindfulness and sleep enhance recovery, ensuring continued resilience and performance.

Merriam-Webster (n.d.) defines *restoration* as:

- Bringing back to a former position or condition (e.g., restoration of peace)

- Restitution of something taken away or lost

- A restoring to an unimpaired or improved condition

In the context of non-living things, restoration refers to returning something to its original state, such as reforesting land or preserving historic buildings. These efforts highlight the importance of intentional actions to repair and maintain what is vital for future generations.

For people, restoration involves replenishing energy, focus, and emotional balance. With constant demands, rest is essential for maintaining health. Activities like nature walks, mindfulness, or creative hobbies help restore calm and clarity. Embracing restoration as a continual process fosters resilience, ensuring individuals can thrive and face new challenges, emerging stronger and renewed.

"As a profession, we can no longer afford to pretend that nursing bullying, incivility, and even violence in the workplace doesn't happen."
Renee Thompson, DNP, CSP, FAAN
CEO and founder, Healthy Workforce Institute

CIVILITY IN THE WORKPLACE

Grit in the workplace is not only about personal resilience and perseverance but also about cultivating civility and respect among colleagues. Civility promotes a supportive environment, encouraging collaboration even in high-stress situations. Practicing patience, empathy, and effective communication are essential aspects of civility. When combined with professionalism and kindness, grit fosters motivation and inspires others, contributing to a more cohesive and productive team.

WHY IT MATTERS

Civility is critical in healthcare, as collaboration, communication, and trust directly impact patient care. In nursing, high-pressure environments demand focus and efficiency. Civility ensures that nurses can collaborate seamlessly under stress, reducing misunderstandings and promoting cooperation. By maintaining civility, nurses create a positive workplace culture that improves team morale and enhances patient outcomes.

PROMOTING RESPECTFUL COMMUNICATION

Respectful communication is essential for civility in nursing. Nurses must engage with colleagues, patients, and healthcare professionals with clarity and empathy. Active listening and avoiding dismissive behaviors ensure effective interactions. Respectful communication fosters an open dialogue where concerns are shared, ideas are discussed, and conflicts are addressed constructively, improving team dynamics and minimizing errors.

MANAGING STRESS AND CONFLICT WITH CIVILITY

Stress and conflict are inevitable but manageable with civility. Conflict management strategies, such as remaining calm, addressing issues promptly, and collaborating for solutions, ensure a productive resolution. Nurses who practice civility focus on solutions, creating a positive environment that reduces tension and fosters resilience and cooperation.

THE ROLE OF LEADERSHIP IN BUILDING CIVILITY

Nurse leaders are pivotal in promoting civility by modeling respect and inclusivity. By setting clear expectations, providing training, and recognizing positive behaviors, leadership creates a culture of civility that improves teamwork and job satisfaction.

THE BENEFITS OF A CIVIL WORKPLACE IN NURSING

A workplace that prioritizes civility benefits nurses, patients, and the healthcare system. Civility shapes the culture and behaviors that drive team success. It reduces burnout, enhances job satisfaction, and fosters a sense of community among nursing teams. When nurses feel respected and supported, they are more engaged and motivated to provide high-quality care. Patients benefit from improved collaboration and better care. Leaders must act swiftly when civility is compromised, as failure to address it can have serious consequences. Civility in nursing is foundational for compassionate, effective healthcare delivery. Addressing incivility requires training, open communication, strong leadership support, and fostering respect and teamwork. A positive work environment improves job satisfaction and patient outcomes, benefiting everyone involved (Weinstein, 2024).

THE HIERARCHY

The hierarchical structure in healthcare creates an oppressive culture, especially for those with less power, affecting relationships between nurses and patients. The "eat your young" mentality, which has been present in nursing for decades, requires a cultural shift. Addressing this issue with diligence is essential for improving retention and fostering a sense of belonging and inclusivity, leading to better patient care and job satisfaction.

FINDING BALANCE

Breaking Down Oppressive Systems

These are the top 10 ways to diffuse oppressive systems in nursing and healthcare:

1. **Create clear policies with clear definitions:**
   Ensure that policies differentiate between bullying, incivility, discrimination, harassment, and other behaviors. Establish a transparent process for handling complaints about disruptive behaviors. Many organizations fail to define this process effectively.

2. **Provide initial and ongoing skill development related to culture and conduct:**
   Review existing educational programs and incorporate content related to culture and conduct. This team approach should include orientation, physician onboarding, nurse residency programs, preceptor programs, and leadership development. Rather than creating new programs, augment current ones with this crucial content.

3. **Incorporate healthy workforce topics as a standing agenda item in all meetings:**
   Embed the principles of a healthy workforce into the organizational culture by making these topics a consistent part of meetings at every level. This approach helps reinforce behavioral expectations, provides ongoing skill development related to professionalism and respect, and fosters a stronger, more cohesive team.

4. Educate new leaders:

Ensure new leaders receive education on addressing disruptive behaviors as part of their orientation. These skills are essential, not "soft," and should be prioritized in their onboarding.

5. Provide ongoing skill development for leaders:

Offer monthly opportunities for leaders to learn how to cultivate a healthy work culture. Topics should include reducing gossip, giving and receiving feedback, and building a trusting culture. Encourage interprofessional leadership teams to engage in conversations about bullying, incivility, burnout, and culture, including HR representatives in these discussions.

6. Be willing to terminate a toxic employee—no matter what:

Support leaders in their efforts to maintain a healthy work environment by allowing them to terminate toxic employees, regardless of the employee's competence, tenure, or revenue generation.

7. Raise awareness:

Educate employees about behaviors that undermine professionalism, respect, and patient safety. Address the normalization of bad behaviors and discriminatory acts, and challenge attitudes such as "that's just the way they are."

8. Engage employees as partners:

Involve the entire team in setting expectations for professional behavior toward one another, new team members, the interprofessional team, and external support staff.

9. Providing ongoing skill development to employees:

Offer employees continuous education, tools, and resources to maintain and enhance a professional, nurturing, and supportive work culture.

10. Create a safe space for open discussions:

Allow teams to have open, nonjudgmental, and nonretaliatory discussions about actions, behaviors, procedures, and policies that are uncivil or oppressive toward staff and patients. End with key takeaways that will reshape culture by incorporating into huddles, staff meetings, and codes of conduct.

BALANCE BREVITIES . . . ACTION STEPS

- Balancing life and work requires mindful prioritization.
- The journey to harmony and balance thrives on self-compassion, grace, and self-forgiveness.
- HNHN (HNHN.org) is a free program that helps healthcare professionals improve holistic self-care.
- Grit is essential for individuals and systems.
- Self-regulation prevents amygdala hijacking, promoting optimal functioning and emotional control.
- Oppressive work environments foster incivility, negatively impacting individuals, systems, and patient care.

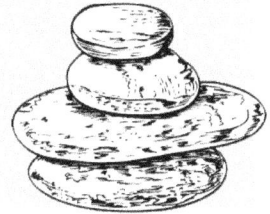

REFERENCES

American Association of Colleges of Nursing. (2021). *The essentials: Core competencies for professional nursing education.* https://www.aacnnursing.org/Portals/0/PDFs/Publications/Essentials-2021.PDF

American Holistic Health Association. (n.d.). *Understanding holistic.* https://ahha.org/understanding-holistic/

American Nurses Association. (2021). *National Commission to Address Racism in Nursing.* https://www.nursingworld.org/practice-policy/workforce/racism-in-nursing/national-commission-to-address-racism-in-nursing?utm_source=chatgpt.com

Bonifacio, R. (2024, Nov. 25). *Prioritizing employee well-being in the workplace: The employer's guide.* Shiftbase. https://www.shiftbase.com/glossary/employee-well-being

Bowen College. (n.d.). *What is holistic health? Understanding the principles and practices.* https://www.bowencollege.com/what-is-holistic-health-understanding-the-principles-and-practices/

Clifton, J., & Harter, J. (2021). *Wellbeing at work: How to build resilient and thriving teams.* Gallup Press.

College of Education at the University of Texas at Austin. (2025). *The two wolves.* https://sites.edb.utexas.edu/resilienceeducation/inspiring-stories/the-two-wolves/#:~:text=One%20wolf%20represents%20fear%2C%20anger,truth%2C%20compassion%20and%20faith.%E2%80%9D

Cuncic, A. (2023). *How to develop and practice self-regulation.* VeryWell Mind. https://www.verywellmind.com/how-you-can-practice-self-regulation-4163536

Duckworth, A. (2016). *Grit: The power of passion and perseverance.* Scribner.

Hampson, S. E., Edmonds, G. W., Barckley, M., Goldberg, L. R., Dubanoski, J. P., & Hillier, T. A. (2016). A big five approach to self-regulation: Personality traits and health trajectories in the Hawaii longitudinal study of personality and health. *Psychology, Health & Medicine, 21*(2), 152–162. https://doi.org/10.1080/13548506.2015.1061676

King, L. M. (2024, Sept. 26). *What is Maslow's Hierarchy of Needs.* WebMD. *https://www.webmd.com/mental-health/what-is-maslow-hierarchy-of-needs*

Merriam-Webster. (n.d.). Restoration. In *Merriam-Webster.com dictionary.* https://www.merriam-webster.com/dictionary/restoration

Sirgy, M. J., & Lee, D. J. (2023). Making the case for work-life balance. In M. J. Sirgy & D. J. Lee, *Work-life balance: HR training for employee personal interventions* (pp. 1–38). Cambridge University Press.

Weinstein, S. M. (2024, Sept. 10). *Leadership's role in shaping workplace culture: Civility as an essential outcome.* HR.com. https://www.hr.com/en/magazines/human_experience_excellence_at_work/september_2024_human_experience_excellence_at_work/leaderships-role-in-shaping-workplace-culture-civi_m0waf4fa.html?utm_source=email&utm_campaign=url&utm_content=leadershipsroleinshapingworkplaceculture%3Acivilityasanessentialoutcome

Willcox, G. (1982). The Feeling Wheel: A tool for expanding awareness of emotions and increasing spontaneity and intimacy. *Transactional Analysis Journal, 12*(4), 274–276. https://doi.org/10.1177/036215378201200411

Wisner, W. (2024, May 30). *Holistic health: A guide to better health and well-being.* https://www.health.com/holistic-health-8652522

Yeow, J., & Martin, R. (2013, October). The role of self-regulation in developing leaders: A longitudinal field experiment. *The Leadership Quarterly, 24*(5), 625–637. https://doi.org/10.1016/j.leaqua.2013.04.004

III

ADAPTIVE SHIFT PLANNING

"Change will not come if we wait for some other person or some other time. We are the ones we've been waiting for. We are the change that we seek."

—Barack Obama, former President of the United States

5

UNDERSTANDING FLEXIBLE SCHEDULING

Sharon M. Weinstein, MS, RN, CRNI-R®, CVP, CSP, FAAN

UNDERSTANDING ADAPTIVE SCHEDULING IN HEALTHCARE: FLEXIBILITY FOR A CHANGING WORKFORCE

Adaptive leaders are ready to pivot and navigate new models by anticipating and embracing change, practicing self-awareness, building trust, and valuing the insights of those within the organization. Nowhere is this more obvious than in the healthcare professions.

Let's face it: The healthcare professions have unique needs, including long hours, emotional resilience, and constant vigilance. The stress of the work environment leads to high burnout rates and recognition of the need to do better. Along comes adaptive or flexible scheduling, an evolving concept in healthcare and an attractive option for both organizations and employees.

Adaptive scheduling is not a single model but a focus on job sharing, shift flexibility, and virtual and part-time work that can accommodate our diverse needs while ensuring the continuity of service delivery. The result is that employees have more control over their working hours, shift patterns, and workload distribution. In healthcare, this means designing schedules that meet the operational needs of hospitals and health systems and align with the personal needs of healthcare professionals. Unlike traditional fixed schedules, adaptive scheduling offers several advantages:

- **Improved work-life integration:** Nurses and other healthcare workers can adjust their schedules to accommodate personal responsibilities, reducing stress and burnout.

- **Enhanced staff retention:** Offering flexibility can increase job satisfaction and reduce turnover, as well as the costs associated with training new employees.

- **Increased patient care quality:** Well-rested, satisfied nurses are more likely to provide attentive, high-quality care.

Adaptive scheduling can be applied to multiple business models, including the hospitality and emergency response spaces, and artificial intelligence (AI)–powered tools can be utilized to create schedules that accommodate nurses' personal and professional needs while maintaining high standards of patient care. Research on flexible scheduling provides nurses and healthcare leaders with insights into the benefits of flexible scheduling and practical strategies for its implementation, ensuring that it meets the needs of the workforce and the organization alike (National Institute for Occupational Safety and Health, 2024; Ray & Pana-Cryan, 2021):

- Working at home increased the likelihood of job stress by 22% and job satisfaction by 65%.

- Taking time off decreased the likelihood of job stress by 56% and days with activity limitations by 24%, and more than doubled the likelihood of job satisfaction.

- Changing one's schedule decreased the likelihood of job stress by 20% and increased job satisfaction by 62%.

Adaptive scheduling models vary widely depending on organizational needs and the specific roles of the healthcare staff. Understanding flexible staffing in healthcare means grasping the concept, strategies, and importance of adjusting staffing levels and schedules to meet fluctuating patient demands, acuity ratios, staff availability, and operational needs. It involves recognizing different staffing models, such as per diem, part time, or float pools, and understanding how these models can reduce burnout, improve job satisfaction, and enhance patient care (Maglalang et al., 2021).

The concept is based on getting the right people in the right place at the right time. Self-scheduling has long been viewed as a critical element of work-life balance and flexibility for nurses. Self-scheduling was first implemented in the 1960s at a hospital in England, with greater adoption in the US in the 1980s. Self-scheduling allows nurses to select their preferred shifts within a scheduled period while meeting specific requirements and parameters, such as weekends or holidays (Gray et al., 2024).

Types of Flexible Scheduling

Job Sharing

Job sharing allows two or more employees to share the responsibilities of one full-time position. In healthcare, this can involve two nurses splitting a single role, each working part time but covering the full-time hours together. This model is beneficial, particularly for healthcare professionals who may want to reduce their working hours due to family commitments, education, or personal health.

Benefits

- Allows nurses to reduce their hours without fully stepping away from their profession

- Provides continuity of care, as two part-time employees can offer combined full-time coverage

- Increases collaboration between job sharers, who must communicate effectively to meet patient needs and ensure patient needs are met

Challenges

- Coordination between job sharers is critical, and lack of communication can lead to gaps in patient care or errors.

- Employers may find matching the correct pairs for job sharing challenging if work styles differ significantly.

Best Practices

- Apply clear communication protocols between job sharers to maintain consistency in patient care.

- Align work schedules to ensure smooth handovers and continuity.

- Assign complementary tasks that make the most of everyone's strengths.

SHIFT FLEXIBILITY

Shift flexibility allows healthcare workers to choose when they work within a set framework. In this model, staff may adhere to a core schedule, but there is flexibility regarding their shifts' start and end times.

Benefits

- Provides nurses autonomy over their schedules, leading to higher job satisfaction and reduced burnout

- Accommodates personal needs without sacrificing coverage

- Reduces absenteeism because nurses can adjust their schedules to meet personal responsibilities instead of calling out

Challenges

- Shift flexibility requires advanced scheduling tools to ensure adequate coverage and avoid conflicts.

- Continuity of care might be affected if shifts are too fragmented or poorly coordinated.

Best Practices

- Implement AI-driven scheduling tools that predict patient volume and match staff availability accordingly.

- Offer clear guidelines for shift swapping to avoid coverage gaps.

- Ensure open communication between nurses and managers to address scheduling conflicts early.

"The pandemic catalyzed a telehealth revolution."
–Byron Carlisle, MSN, RN, CCRN-K, SCRN
Director of Neuroscience Services, UT Southwestern Medical Center

---

VIRTUAL NURSING

Virtual nursing is a viable solution to healthcare staffing challenges, especially in creating more flexible work options. By leveraging technology, virtual nursing enables registered nurses to work remotely, providing patient care support through telehealth platforms, patient monitoring systems, and digital communications. This model enhances staffing flexibility, allowing nurses to work from diverse locations and roles, from patient education to discharge planning and monitoring, without needing to be physically present onsite. The benefits are abundant (Schmidt, 2023)!

Benefits

- Expands the healthcare workforce beyond geographic limitations, allowing facilities to tap into a broader talent pool, including nurses who want to reduce their hours or retire due to possible physical limitations

- Helps healthcare systems in rural or underserved areas where staffing shortages are more pronounced

- Enables virtual nurses to offer 24/7 support and oversight of new nurses

- Alleviates burnout by offering nurses alternative work environments that reduce the physical strain associated with bedside care by focusing on specific patient care aspects like monitoring and follow-ups

- Ensures more consistent, quality care across shifts, easing the workload for onsite staff

- Improves patient outcomes through better monitoring and rapid responses to patient needs, especially when integrated with intelligent technology

- Allows supporting multiple hospitals within a system and streamlines repetitive tasks like appointment scheduling and documentation

Challenges

- Must provide robust and secure telehealth systems alongside a reliable IT infrastructure to function effectively.

- Ensuring the human connection may be an issue— patients may initially feel disconnected.

- Maintaining privacy and data security is crucial because virtual nursing increases potential cyber risks and requires strict adherence to data protection standards.

- Navigating licensure across state lines can be complicated, as virtual nurses may serve patients in multiple locations.

Best Practices

- Plan carefully, invest in high-quality telehealth technology, and ensure robust cybersecurity measures to protect patient information.

- Ensure seamless collaboration and training for virtual nurses and onsite staff.

- Define clear roles and responsibilities for virtual nurses to prevent overlapping and confusion with onsite staff.

- Establish reliable communication protocols and a channel with in-person care teams and patients.

Adopting a phased approach to virtual nursing can help organizations adjust and refine their processes. Starting with lower-risk, high-impact areas like patient monitoring allows healthcare systems to evaluate and address potential issues before scaling up. Seeking patient feedback is also critical, as this can guide improvements and ensure that virtual care meets the patients' needs. With strategic implementation, virtual nursing can be a powerful tool in addressing flexible staffing needs and enhancing the overall quality of care. As virtual nursing grows, organization leaders respond by formalizing competencies and potential certifications.

"Imagine if the same virtual nurse who cared for you in the hospital performed a virtual visit after discharge or was your hospital-to-home nurse and connected with your primary care provider for a warm handoff. This future helps us add tremendous value to those we serve. It moves nurses into the space of holistic care coordination as outlined in the IOM: Future of Nursing 2030."

—Anne Antrum, DNP, RN
Systemwide Chief Nursing Officer, Cone Health

PART-TIME WORK

Part-time work reduces the workload for healthcare professionals who may need more time but cannot commit to full-time hours. In nursing, this can involve working a set number of hours per week on a predictable or flexible schedule. Part-time roles can be valuable for nurses nearing retirement, those pursuing further education, or those balancing family obligations.

Benefits

- Retains skilled nurses who might otherwise leave the profession due to an inability to commit to full-time work

- Reduces burnout by limiting nurses' hours in high-stress environments

- Provides a pipeline for recruiting full-time nurses, as part-time employees may eventually transition to full-time roles

Challenges

- Staffing part-time workers can create logistical challenges, as more employees are needed to cover the same number of hours.

- Part-time workers may have less continuity with patients, potentially affecting care outcomes.

Best Practices

- Clearly define part-time roles to ensure consistent coverage and workload distribution.

- Pair part-time workers with full-time staff to ensure continuous patient care. Regularly reassess part-time schedules to ensure they align with the organization's needs and the employees' preferences.

MONITORING AND ADJUSTING SCHEDULES

Adaptive scheduling requires continuous monitoring and adjustments to ensure it remains effective for staff and patients. This can be achieved through several methods:

- **Data-driven decision-making:** Healthcare organizations should collect data on staff satisfaction, absenteeism, turnover rates, and patient outcomes to assess the success of flexible scheduling. Advanced scheduling tools that use AI and machine learning can help predict patient needs, adjust staffing levels, and recommend optimal schedules based on real-time data.

- **Regular feedback from staff:** Engaging nurses and other healthcare workers in regular feedback sessions ensures the scheduling system meets their needs. This feedback can also identify areas with more flexibility or highlight emerging issues, such as burnout or staffing gaps.

- **Compliance monitoring:** Ensuring flexible scheduling models adhere to labor laws, union agreements, and other legal requirements is critical. For example, regulations on overtime, break periods, and maximum shift lengths must be observed. Automated scheduling systems can help flag potential compliance issues and prevent violations before they occur.

- **Adjustments based on patient care metrics:** Patient care outcomes should always be a priority in healthcare scheduling. If flexible schedules are leading to issues with patient care, such as delayed response times or fragmented care, adjustments must be made. This could involve refining shift patterns, improving communication between part-time and full-time staff, or increasing the use of float pools to cover high-demand periods.

FINDING BALANCE

Let's ADAPT!

The acronym ADAPT showcases critical components of adaptive scheduling in the healthcare space:

- **A: Assess needs**
  Evaluate the needs of both patients and staff regularly. This includes understanding peak times for patient care, staff availability, and special requirements (e.g., for high-acuity patients). Accurate assessments help create a responsive schedule.

- **D: Data-driven decisions**
  Utilize data analytics to inform scheduling practices. Analyze patient flow, staff performance, and resource utilization to optimize schedules. This approach helps anticipate demand and reduce waiting times, enhancing care delivery.

- **A: Agile practices**
  Embrace flexibility in scheduling. Allow for last-minute adjustments and changes based on real-time needs, such as unexpected patient admissions or staff absences. Agile practices ensure that resources are allocated efficiently, adapting to changing circumstances.

- **P: Prioritize well-being**
  Focus on the well-being of healthcare staff by considering their work-life balance in scheduling. Incorporate preferences and ensure adequate breaks. Prioritizing staff well-being reduces burnout and improves job satisfaction, improving patient care (International Council of Nurses, 2021).

- **T: Team collaboration**
  Foster open communication and collaboration among team members. Involve staff in the scheduling process, encouraging feedback and input. Collaborative scheduling builds a sense of ownership and accountability, enhancing team dynamics and operational efficiency.

By implementing the ADAPT principles in adaptive scheduling, healthcare organizations can improve operational efficiency, enhance staff satisfaction, and ultimately deliver better patient care. Continuously revisiting and refining these strategies will help ensure their ongoing effectiveness in an ever-changing healthcare environment.

Flexible and adaptive scheduling is a powerful tool for healthcare organizations seeking to improve nurse well-being, reduce burnout, and maintain high standards of patient care. By offering job sharing, shift flexibility, and part-time work options, healthcare facilities can accommodate the diverse needs of their workforce. However, successful implementation requires careful planning, data-driven monitoring, and ongoing adjustments to meet the evolving demands of both staff and patients. With the right approach, flexible scheduling can enhance the resilience and adaptability of healthcare organizations in a rapidly changing industry.

LEGAL AND LOGISTICAL CONSIDERATIONS

Careful consideration of labor laws and logistical planning ensures compliance and maintains optimal staffing levels.

LEGAL CONSIDERATIONS

- **Labor laws and fair scheduling:** Flexible scheduling must comply with federal, state, and local labor laws. Some states have "fair workweek" laws mandating advance notice of schedules, limits on last-minute changes, and predictable shifts. Employers need to stay updated on these regulations to avoid penalties.

- **Overtime and minimum wage:** Under the US Fair Labor Standards Act (FLSA), non-exempt employees must receive overtime pay at 1.5 times their regular rate for hours worked over 40 in a workweek. Flexible scheduling must be designed to prevent unintended overtime and to comply with both federal and state wage laws (US Department of Labor, n.d.).

- **Overtime exceptions and exemptions:** Exempt employees, typically salaried professionals, are not entitled to overtime under FLSA (US Department of Labor, n.d.). However, healthcare employees may have specific exemptions based on their roles. Correctly classify workers to ensure legal compliance with overtime pay requirements.

- **Breaks and rest periods:** States often require specific breaks and meal periods. Flexible schedules must ensure employees receive mandated rest breaks and meal periods, even working non-standard hours.

- **Union contracts:** Flexible scheduling must align with existing collective bargaining agreements for unionized employees. Negotiations with unions may be necessary to change scheduling practices.

- **Work-life balance and compliance with family leave:** Flexible scheduling should be compatible with family and medical leave policies. Employers must allow employees eligible for FMLA or other state-mandated leaves to take time off without penalty.

MANDATORY OVERTIME

A word about mandatory overtime: In discussions with nurses face to face, mandatory overtime remains a concern, despite legislation passed by Congress and applauded by the American Nurses Association (2024). While a quick fix to the nursing shortage, the result is a negative impact on nurses and patient care. Chronic or ongoing mandatory overtime affects nurses and those they care for (Deering, 2023). While many US states have enacted laws regarding compulsory overtime for nurses, others have not. We cannot allow the demands for productivity in any workspace to clash with team members' personal lives. See the Appendix for more on mandatory overtime.

LOGISTICAL CONSIDERATIONS

The next chapter addresses the implementation of flexible scheduling in depth. For now, consider:

- **Demand forecasting:** Use data analytics to anticipate patient volume and staffing needs across different times and seasons. This ensures staffing levels are consistently met without excessive reliance on last-minute changes or overtime.

- **Shift bidding and self-scheduling tools:** Implement software that enables shift bidding or self-scheduling, allowing employees to choose shifts that align with their availability. These systems empower employees while ensuring that all required shifts are covered.

- **Cross-training:** Cross-train staff members in multiple roles so they can cover different functions. This reduces the need for additional staff and enables more fluid scheduling.

- **Core and flex staffing models:** Implement a core group of full-time staff for essential hours, complemented by a flexible pool of part-time or per-diem workers who can cover peak times. This allows organizations to meet fluctuating demands without overstaffing.

- **Automated scheduling software:** Use scheduling software that considers employee preferences, labor laws, and overtime regulations. Such software can prevent scheduling conflicts, track overtime, and ensure compliance while accommodating employee flexibility.

- **On-call policies and shift swaps:** Establish on-call and shift swap policies that allow employees to adjust schedules while ensuring complete coverage. Clear guidelines help prevent last-minute gaps and reduce staff burnout.

By carefully aligning flexible scheduling with legal requirements and utilizing practical scheduling tools and policies, healthcare organizations can provide staff with greater work-life balance without compromising patient care.

"When we prioritize our people, we invest in the foundation of our healthcare system."

–Christine Pabico
Senior Director, Pathway to Excellence Program, ANCC

BALANCE BREVITIES . . . ACTION STEPS

Here are four action steps for re-imagining adaptive scheduling and your care model to enhance flexibility and maintain balance:

1. Identify the conversations you should be having internally about adaptive scheduling.

2. Evaluate potential organizational interest in the available options.

3. Assess and determine your capacity, including workforce, technology, and finances, plus scaling.

4. Consider how to measure and evaluate the success of your adaptive scheduling process.

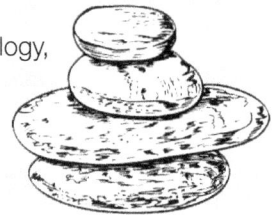

REFERENCES

American Nurses Association. (2024, May 7). *ANA commends introduction of the Nurse Overtime and Patient Safety Act.* https://www.nursingworld.org/news/news-releases/2024/ana-commends-introduction-of-the-nurse-overtime-and-patient-safety-act/

Deering, M. (2023, Oct. 3). Understanding mandatory overtime for nurses: Which states enforce mandatory overtime? *NurseJournal.* https://nursejournal.org/resources/mandatory-overtime-for-nurses/

Gray, S., Ragusa Morris, M., & Bowie, D. (2024). The power of self-scheduling: Frontline nurses' insights and perspectives to achieve staffing flexibility. *Nurse Leader, 22*(4), 438–444. https://doi.org/10.1016/j.mnl.2023.11.012

International Council of Nurses. (2021). *ICN policy brief: The global nursing shortage and nurse retention.* https://www.icn.ch/sites/default/files/inline-files/ICN%20Policy%20Brief_Nurse%20Shortage%20and%20Retention.pdf

Maglalang, D. D., Sorensen, G., Hopcia, K., Hashimoto, D. M., Katigbak, C., Pandey, S., Takeuchi, D., & Sabbath, E. L. (2021). Job and family demands and burnout among healthcare workers: The moderating role of workplace flexibility. *SSM – Population Health, 14,* 100802. https://doi.org/10.1016/j.ssmph.2021.100802

National Institute for Occupational Safety and Health. (2024, April 22). *Quality of worklife questionnaire.* https://www.cdc.gov/niosh/stress/worklife-question/?CDC_AAref_Val=https://www.cdc.gov/niosh/topics/stress/qwlquest.html

Ray, T. K., & Pana-Cryan, R. (2021). Work flexibility and work-related well-being. *International Journal of Environmental Research & Public Health, 18*(6), 3254. https://doi.org/10.3390/ijerph18063254

Schmidt, A. (2023, Sept. 4). *Virtual nursing: What it is, and why we need it.* Advisory Board. https://www.advisory.com/topics/nursing/2023/09/virtual-nursing-what-it-is-and-why-we-need-it

US Department of Labor. (n.d.). *Overtime.* https://www.dol.gov/general/topic/workhours/overtime#:~:text=For%20covered%2C%20nonexempt%20employees%2C%20the,from%20the%20elaws%20FLSA%20Advisor

"Nurses are a unique kind. They have this insatiable need to care for others, which is both their greatest strength and fatal flaw."

—Jean Watson, nurse theorist, Caring Science

6

IMPLEMENTING FLEXIBLE SCHEDULING

Sharon M. Weinstein, MS, RN, CRNI-R®, CVP, CSP, FAAN

Nurses, who often endure long hours, high patient loads, and the emotional strain of caring for critically ill patients, need relief. These hurdles contribute to burnout and high turnover rates, making it challenging for healthcare organizations to maintain stable staffing. Flexible scheduling offers a much-needed solution, empowering nurses to select or adjust their shifts, cater to personal needs, and significantly reduce stress. This approach benefits nurses' well-being and enhances job satisfaction, reducing turnover rates and improving patient care.

In addition to improving personal well-being, flexible scheduling helps address absenteeism, improves retention rates, and boosts job satisfaction. Flexible scheduling can lead to higher productivity, fewer errors, and improved patient outcomes, as nurses are more likely to be engaged and focused when work-life balance is prioritized.

THE CASE FOR FLEXIBLE SCHEDULING

Implementing flexible staffing goes beyond theory; it involves actively implementing these strategies and recognizing the positive and negative consequences (Lee & Chang, 2022; Ray & Pana-Cryan, 2021).

This includes:

- Creating dynamic staffing plans that adapt to patient volumes

- Leveraging technology and predictive analytics to forecast staffing needs

- Negotiating with staff to accommodate preferences for work hours, shift lengths, or remote options when possible

- Overcoming union rules, budget constraints, or administrative resistance

- Monitoring outcomes and adjusting based on feedback and changing circumstances

The difference is that understanding involves the "what" and "why" of flexible staffing while implementing focuses on the "how" and ensuring its success in day-to-day operations.

Flexible scheduling in healthcare is increasingly recognized as a solution to the industry's staffing challenges, burnout rates, and retention issues. By shifting away from rigid schedules, healthcare organizations can improve staff well-being and enhance patient care. The success of flexible scheduling hinges on thoughtful planning, monitoring, and, most importantly, continual adjustments to balance organizational needs and staff preferences. This ongoing commitment to improvement keeps everyone, including administrators, engaged and committed to the cause, ensuring the best outcomes for all.

KEY CONSIDERATIONS

Despite the clear benefits, implementing flexible scheduling in healthcare is challenging. It requires navigating legal regulations, logistical complexities, and potential resistance from both staff and management. To ensure a successful transition, organizations must consider the following factors:

- **Legal and regulatory compliance:** Flexible scheduling must comply with labor laws, including overtime, break times, and maximum shift lengths. Unions and collective bargaining agreements may have specific provisions about working hours and shift patterns that must be addressed.

- **Technology and tools:** Advanced scheduling tools, such as artificial intelligence (AI)–driven platforms, can facilitate flexible scheduling by predicting staffing needs and automating shift assignments based on nurse availability and patient demand. These tools can help avoid overstaffing or understaffing, allowing nurses to request shifts or swap with colleagues easily.

- **Nurse preferences and availability:** Implementing flexible scheduling involves understanding staff preferences. Surveys or focus groups can help identify needs, such as self-scheduling, compressed workweeks, or shift swapping. Incorporating these preferences into the scheduling model is crucial for gaining buy-in and ensuring the system meets nurses' needs.

- **Shift work disorder:** Shift work disorder (SWD) affects many professionals working nontraditional hours, leading to sleep disturbances and fatigue. This misalignment of the body's circadian rhythm increases the risk of physical and mental health issues, including cardiovascular problems, depression, and reduced cognitive function. To combat SWD, it's important to maintain a consistent sleep schedule, limit caffeine intake (including energy drinks), and create a restful environment. Regular shift rotations and better scheduling practices can help manage symptoms and promote well-being. For more on managing SWD and fatigue, see the Appendix.

- **Patient care considerations:** While nurses' flexibility is essential, patient care remains the top priority. Schedules must ensure adequate coverage during peak hours and high patient loads and maintain continuity of care.

FOLLOW THE STEPS

The critical steps of deploying flexible scheduling in an organization are as follows:

1. **Conduct a needs assessment:** Before changing scheduling, organizations should assess staff needs and patient care requirements. This could include collecting data on current scheduling challenges, understanding legal and logistical constraints, and gathering input from nurses on their preferences for flexible work arrangements.

2. **Develop a pilot program:** Launching a pilot program allows healthcare organizations to test flexible scheduling models before full implementation. A small-scale trial in one unit or department can help identify potential issues, such as gaps in coverage or conflicts with patient care. The pilot program should also include clear metrics for success, such as nursing satisfaction, retention rates, and patient outcomes.

3. **Invest in technology:** AI-powered scheduling tools automate complex processes, optimizing schedules by analyzing patient volumes, staffing levels, and preferences. Nurses can view shifts, request changes, or swap, ensuring adequate staffing.

4. **Provide training and support:** Successful implementation requires clear communication and training for nurses and managers. They must understand the new scheduling system, shift requests, and patient care maintenance, with a focus on both technical aspects and cultural change.

5. **Monitor and adjust schedules:** Implementing flexible scheduling requires ongoing monitoring of key performance indicators like staff satisfaction and patient outcomes, with regular nurse feedback to identify areas for improvement and adjustments.

6. **Address resistance:** Resistance to change is common in scheduling. Healthcare leaders should involve stakeholders early, including nurses, to gain buy-in and address concerns about control and productivity.

If the "how" is overwhelming, consider a design thinking approach.

Design Thinking

The 4Ws and Design Thinking

Flexible staffing in healthcare is more than a buzzword; it's an essential strategy for creating resilient healthcare environments. By aligning staffing resources with patient demand and staff preferences, healthcare organizations can enhance patient care and employee satisfaction.

Implementing flexible staffing requires a thoughtful approach and applying the *4Ws,* a process attributed to Jeanne Liedtka (2018). **What Is, What If, What Wows,** and **What Works** can guide leaders in designing and executing effective staffing strategies through observation, using different lenses, brainstorming, and assessing the solution (Readinger & Weinstein, 2022).

What Is? Understanding the Current State of Staffing

Before implementing flexible staffing, it's crucial to understand the baseline: what the current staffing model looks like, where gaps exist, and how those gaps impact patient care. Traditional staffing models often rely on fixed schedules, leading to inefficiencies, staff burnout, and variability in patient care quality.

In the What Is? phase, ask key questions:

- **What are the staffing needs?** Understand the fluctuating demands of patient care, including peak times and low periods.
- **What challenges do staff face?** Acknowledge issues like burnout, work-life balance, and dissatisfaction with rigid schedules.

This phase is all about gathering data. Use surveys, patient volume trends, and staffing metrics to depict the current state. Flexible staffing must be built on a foundation of real-world needs, not assumptions.

What If? Exploring Potential Solutions

Once you understand the current state, the next step is to explore what could change: What if we implemented new staffing models? This phase involves considering different options, some of which may be unconventional or creative.

Key considerations in the What If? phase include:

- What if we shifted to self-scheduling? Allowing staff to choose their shifts could improve morale and reduce turnover.

- What if we created a float pool? A dedicated team of staff who can fill in across different units can add flexibility.

- What if we used predictive analytics? Leveraging data to forecast patient demand and align staffing can minimize over- or understaffing.

- What if we introduced part-time or per diem positions? Offering nontraditional working hours could attract staff who might otherwise leave the workforce.

- What if the staff completely designed schedules? Would giving employees complete control over their schedules lead to higher job satisfaction and retention?

Imagination and flexibility are critical in this phase. Leaders should collaborate with staff, encourage feedback, and brainstorm solutions challenging the status quo. These "What if" questions push the boundaries of traditional thinking, inspiring new approaches to create more flexible, worker-centric schedules in healthcare.

What Wows? Designing an Impactful Flexible Staffing Model

What Wows? is an opportunity to create small-scale models or prototypes to test possible solutions and determine what would wow, given the investment of time, talent, and dollars. The What Wows? phase is about creating a solution that works, excites the organization, and improves outcomes. This step requires integrating the best ideas from the What If? phase and building an innovative, sustainable, and beneficial staffing model for staff and patients.

A flexible staffing model that "wows" might include:

- **AI-powered scheduling tools:** Implement advanced technology that provides real-time visibility into staffing needs and allows for dynamic adjustments.

- **Cross-training programs:** These programs equip staff with the skills to work across multiple units, offering flexibility in staffing while expanding professional development.

- **On-demand staffing:** Apps allow nurses and other healthcare professionals to pick up shifts as needed, using a mobile platform like gig-economy models.

- **Flexible shift lengths and job-sharing options:** Offering staff the option to work shorter or split shifts increases satisfaction and retention.

The goal is to go beyond incremental improvements—aim for changes that dramatically enhance operational efficiency and work-life balance for staff, leading to a "wow" effect for employees and patients.

What Works? Implementing and Sustaining Flexible Staffing

What Works? refers to identifying practical, feasible, and scalable solutions that have been tested and refined. When applied to retention models in healthcare, this phase focuses on implementing strategies that have proven to effectively improve staff retention, increase job satisfaction, and reduce turnover. This phase involves implementing theory while ensuring the system is sustainable and adaptable.

Key components in the What Works? phase include:

- **Pilot programs:** Start small by testing the new staffing models in one or two departments. Gather data on what works and what doesn't before scaling up.

- **Engaging stakeholders:** Communication is crucial during implementation. Involve department heads, HR, and the staff in refining the model. Transparency fosters trust and cooperation.

- **Technology integration:** Ensure that the technology used to support flexible staffing—whether AI-driven scheduling tools, mobile apps, or analytics platforms—is user-friendly and accessible to all staff.

- **Monitoring and feedback loops:** Monitor key metrics such as staff satisfaction, patient outcomes, and cost-effectiveness. Implement feedback loops where staff can share concerns or suggest improvements.

- **Adapt and evolve:** Flexible staffing models should remain adaptable. As needs change, be prepared to adjust policies, introduce new technologies, or rethink aspects of the program.

Sustaining flexible staffing requires constant evaluation. What works today may not work tomorrow, especially as patient volumes fluctuate, technology evolves, and staff needs change.

MONITORING AND ADJUSTING SCHEDULES

Once flexible scheduling is implemented, ongoing monitoring is essential to ensure it delivers the desired outcomes. Monitoring should focus on several key areas:

- **Staff satisfaction:** Regular surveys or one-on-one check-ins should be conducted to assess how nurses feel about the flexibility of their schedules. High satisfaction levels indicate the system is working, while any concerns can help identify where tweaks may be necessary.

- **Coverage and patient care:** Review patient care metrics, such as response times and continuity of care, to ensure that flexible scheduling isn't leading to gaps in coverage. Any issues with patient care should prompt a review and adjustment of schedules.

- **Compliance:** Review schedules regularly to ensure compliance with labor laws and union agreements. Automated scheduling tools can help by flagging potential violations before they become an issue.

- **Workload distribution:** Ensure that workloads remain evenly distributed among staff. Some flexible scheduling models can unintentionally overburden certain nurses while underutilizing others, so regular reviews are critical.

By continually monitoring and adjusting schedules based on feedback and performance metrics, healthcare organizations can ensure that flexible scheduling remains beneficial to nurses and effective in maintaining high standards of patient care.

BEST PRACTICES

Implementing flexible scheduling requires best practices focused on sustainability and scalability. Using the design thinking approach, healthcare organizations can adapt to evolving needs while ensuring long-term operational resilience and employee satisfaction. A tailored strategy based on the 4Ws—understanding the current state, imagining solutions, creating models, and sustaining them—ensures that flexible staffing benefits staff well-being, patient care, and operational efficiency. This approach transforms flexible staffing into a strategic, future-ready healthcare solution.

Addressing Resistance

"First and foremost, I believe in flexible working. It is important that employers appreciate employees' work-life balance and give them flexibility to work around their personal lives."
—Sir Richard Branson, Virgin Group

Cultural and Operational Resistance

Cultural resistance stems from ingrained beliefs, behaviors, and expectations within the workforce. It can arise from staff, managers, or leadership and is often shaped by long-standing industry norms, such as:

- **Traditionalism and the status quo:** Healthcare has historically operated on fixed, rigid scheduling systems with predictable shifts such as 12-hour blocks or strict day and night shifts.

- **Fear of reduced control:** Managers and supervisors with significant control over schedules often resist flexible staffing because they perceive a loss of authority.

- **Generational differences:** Different generations of workers may be more accepting of flexible staffing (see Chapter 10 for more on generational differences).

- **Union and labor negotiations:** In unionized environments, collective bargaining agreements often lock in rigid scheduling practices that can be difficult to change.

Is it time for a mindset change?

"I resist change in things that I feel comfortable with and that I'm used to."
—Dennis Quaid, actor

OPERATIONAL RESISTANCE: SYSTEMS, LOGISTICS, AND RESOURCES

While cultural resistance focuses on attitudes and beliefs, *operational resistance* deals with the practical or impractical hurdles of transforming existing systems. Some of those hurdles include:

- **Inadequate technology:** Organizations may lack the technological infrastructure to effectively support flexible staffing. Scheduling software, predictive analytics, and mobile platforms are crucial for dynamically adjusting staffing levels based on real-time data, yet many institutions still rely on manual scheduling methods.

  - *Challenge:* This is a nightmare without the right technology; barriers might be software solutions, outdated IT systems, and budgetary constraints.

- **Complexity of managing diverse needs:** Flexible staffing involves balancing patients' needs, staff preferences, and regulatory requirements, such as nurse-to-patient ratios. The complexity of ensuring adequate coverage, skill mix, and compliance with regulations creates operational challenges that may deter organizations from fully embracing flexibility.

  - *Challenge:* Varying schedules and shifts require detailed oversight and continuous adjustment, possibly straining human resources and management teams. There is a fear of gaps in coverage.

- **Training and skillset distribution:** Flexible staffing requires cross-training staff to work in multiple units or perform various roles. Without appropriate training, staff might feel unprepared or overwhelmed by the shifting demands, leading to safety concerns.

  - *Challenge:* Investing in cross-training can be resource-intensive. Some staff may resist cross-training, seeing it as a burden rather than an opportunity for development.

- **Budget constraints:** Implementing flexible staffing often involves additional costs—investments in technology, training, and compensation for staff who fill in during high-demand periods. The perceived cost of implementation may lead to resistance.

  - *Challenge:* Budget concerns create barriers with leadership focused on short-term costs over long-term gains in employee satisfaction and quality of care.

OVERCOMING RESISTANCE: STRATEGIES FOR SUCCESS

Implementing flexible staffing in healthcare often requires overcoming significant cultural and operational resistance. To address these challenges effectively, a multifaceted approach is necessary. Here are key strategies to consider:

- **Education and communication:** Leadership must communicate the benefits of flexible staffing, emphasizing improvements in operational efficiency, work-life balance, and patient outcomes. Engaging staff in open discussions about how flexibility can reduce burnout, improve job satisfaction, and enhance the quality of care can help shift attitudes toward these changes.

- **Engaging staff in solution design:** Involving healthcare workers in designing and implementing flexible staffing systems can reduce resistance. Allowing staff to contribute ideas and voice concerns helps create staffing models that meet their needs and those of the patients. This collaborative approach fosters a sense of ownership and acceptance.

- **Phased implementation:** A gradual, phased approach to rolling out flexible staffing allows time for adjustments and learning. Start with pilot programs in specific departments to evaluate how flexible systems perform. This enables healthcare organizations to identify and address potential issues before scaling the model across the institution.

- **Investment in technology and training:** Successful flexible staffing relies on investing in the right tools, such as scheduling software and cross-training programs for staff. Technology can simplify the scheduling process, making accommodating last-minute changes or shift swaps easier. Cross-training ensures staff are prepared to work in multiple roles as needed, improving flexibility without compromising care.

- **Union collaboration and negotiation:** Engaging with unions early in the planning process is crucial to addressing concerns related to job security, compensation, and working conditions. Collaborating with union leaders helps healthcare organizations design flexible staffing models that benefit both staff and the organization, ensuring a smoother implementation.

- **Highlighting long-term benefits:** Leaders must emphasize the long-term advantages of flexible staffing, including reduced turnover, improved employee well-being, and enhanced patient care. Demonstrating how these benefits positively impact the organization's reputation and bottom line can help alleviate concerns over potential short-term disruptions or initial costs.

Implementing flexible staffing in healthcare requires a comprehensive approach to overcome cultural and operational resistance. By fostering collaboration, investing in technology and training, and emphasizing long-term benefits, healthcare organizations can create flexible staffing models that improve patient care and employee satisfaction. Flexibility is no longer optional in today's healthcare system; it's essential for meeting the evolving needs of both staff and patients.

FINDING BALANCE

The FLEX Framework for Implementing Flexible Staffing

The FLEX framework captures the essential elements for successful flexible staffing in healthcare:

- **F: Foster communication**

  Encourage open dialogue about staff scheduling needs and preferences. Regularly check in with team members for feedback and suggestions. Clear communication helps create schedules that balance both personal and professional needs.

- **L: Leverage technology**

  Use scheduling software that enables easy adjustments and real-time updates. Technology can help with shift swaps, track availability, and streamline scheduling, reducing administrative burdens.

- **E: Emphasize work-life balance**

  Recognize the importance of work-life balance for staff. Implement flexible policies, such as part-time options, shift rotations, and adaptable hours, to accommodate personal commitments. Supporting balance can improve job satisfaction and reduce turnover.

- **X: eXplore innovative models**

  Be open to exploring new scheduling approaches, such as compressed workweeks, self-scheduling, or rotational shifts. Experiment with different models to determine what works best for your team and healthcare setting, which will improve morale and patient care.

By applying the FLEX principles to staffing, healthcare organizations can create a more adaptable, efficient, and satisfied workforce. The result? A flexible staffing system that supports both the well-being of employees and the delivery of high-quality care.

BALANCE BREVITIES . . . ACTION STEPS

Here are four action steps to summarize flexible staffing:

1. Adapt to demand.

2. Empower employees.

3. Cross-train for coverage.

4. Look for scalable solutions.

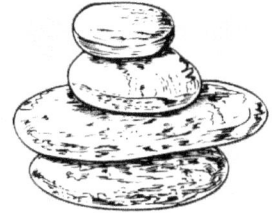

REFERENCES

Lee, H.-F., & Chang, Y.-J. (2022, December). The effects of work satisfaction and work flexibility on burnout in nurses. *Journal Of Nursing Research, 30*(6), E240. https://www.doi.org/10.1097/Jnr.0000000000000522

Liedtka, J. (2018, September–October). Why design thinking works. *Harvard Business Review,* 96(5), 72–79. https://hbr.org/2018/09/why-design-thinking-works

Ray, T. K., & Pana-Cryan, R. (2021). Work flexibility and work-related well-being. *International Journal of Environmental Research and Public Health*, 18(6), 3254. https://www.doi.org/10.3390/ijerph18063254

Readinger, D., & Weinstein, S. (2022) *Think differently: 18 strategies to fix broken thinking.* SMW Group.

IV

MENTAL HEALTH MATTERS

"If you want others to be happy, practice compassion. If you want to be happy, practice compassion."

—Dalai Lama, founder, Mind and Body Institute

7

MENTAL HEALTH IN THE HEALTHCARE PROFESSIONS

Marla J. Vannucci, PhD; Monica Holliday, PsyD

Decades of research highlight specific challenges in maintaining well-being amidst daily pressures and organizational demands. This discussion delves into mental health issues, protective factors against burnout, and resources to support healthcare professionals amid systemic changes.

THE STRUGGLE IS REAL

According to Cranage and Foster (2022), healthcare workers face challenges across four categories: consumer, colleague, role, and organization. Consumer challenges include patient interactions, demands of patient care, and observing suffering, while colleague challenges involve relationships with peers and supervisors, including incivility. Role-related issues involve workload, pace, safety issues, and time management, and organizational challenges include job security, staffing, and compensation.

We can imagine these four types of challenges as the four corners of a square, with your well-being inside it. Feeling overwhelmed in one, two, or even all four of these job aspects will cause the square to shift out of shape, and the more challenges you face, the harder it is to pull the square back into shape. If you struggle to set boundaries or prioritize personal needs, this may also increase the difficulty of maintaining your square's shape. When your square loses its shape, you are at risk for burnout.

Burnout is pervasive, and if left unchecked, it can lead to depression. Signs of burnout are often normalized, making it difficult for healthcare professionals to access support. When burnout leads to depression, this may manifest in feelings of hopelessness, low self-worth, and reduced interest in activities once enjoyed.

The American Nurses Foundation (2025) surveyed mental health and wellness among nurses, revealing that over half of the participants reported burnout symptoms. Despite this high level of burnout, two-thirds of the participants had not accessed mental health support, citing lack of time or financial resources as key barriers. The stigma surrounding mental health concerns was also a significant factor, with 56% of participants reporting that they experienced stigma related to mental health issues. See Chapters 3 and 4 for more details on creating a supportive work environment and promoting work/life balance.

The COVID-19 pandemic exacerbated the issue of burnout among healthcare workers. Nigam et al. (2023) found that 46% of healthcare professionals reported burnout after the pandemic, compared to 32% before. Anxiety and PTSD rates have also skyrocketed since the beginning of the pandemic. The mental and physical demands involved in managing personal safety and attending to patient care increased the strain on healthcare professionals, leading to higher rates of mental health concerns overall.

SUICIDE PREVENTION AND EDUCATION

Some reports suggest that the risk for suicide is three to five times higher for healthcare workers than in the general population. Women, emergency responders, early career professionals, and other frontline workers are most at risk. Exposure to pain and loss, caring for severely ill or injured patients, stressful workloads, and lack of control over clinical outcomes are contributing factors (Hill et al., 2022; Letvak et al., 2012; Maharaj et al., 2019).

Education and prevention programs aim to address this critical threat to well-being, and healthcare workers must know the warning signs of suicide and appropriate responses. Risk factors—including those associated with pandemics, signs/signals of suicide, and debunked misconceptions—as well as specific recommended interventions can be found in the Appendix.

WORKPLACE FACTORS

The Dr. Lorna Breen Healthcare Provider Protection Act (2022) was groundbreaking in dedicating significant federal funding to support evidence-based mental health and suicide-prevention programs and services for healthcare providers.

According to the World Health Organization (2024), employers and policymakers hold a moral obligation to implement a "duty of care" by creating safe, healthy work environments and addressing factors that lead to or exacerbate mental health issues in the healthcare workforce. Suboptimal staff-to-patient ratios threaten quality care, heighten intensity and pressure, and exacerbate fatigue and burnout.

COMPASSION FATIGUE

While burnout is not unique to the helping professions and can occur in any industry or work environment, compassion fatigue distinctly impacts those in helping positions. *Compassion fatigue* manifests as physical, emotional, and spiritual exhaustion associated with repeated exposure to patient suffering. The caring and compassion we need to be effective healthcare professionals also makes us vulnerable to fatigue. Like burnout, compassion fatigue is more likely to occur when work conditions are poor and can lead to mood symptoms like depression and anxiety or physical symptoms like poor sleep or gastrointestinal issues. See Table 7.1 for symptoms of compassion fatigue.

Healthcare workers must prioritize self-care. When asked about their emotional health, 32% of nurses with less than 10 years of experience validated that they are "not emotionally healthy" or "not at all emotionally healthy" (American Nurses Association,

2023). According to Adams et al. (2006), four factors that make us vulnerable to compassion fatigue are having our own trauma experiences, poor self-care, inability to control work demands or stressors, and lack of satisfaction in our work. The COVID-19 pandemic set the stage for compassion fatigue; with self-care a low priority or inaccessible due to the global health crisis, many professionals left the field.

Table 7.1   Symptoms of Compassion Fatigue

Work-Related	Physical	Emotional
Fear, avoidance of specific patients	Headaches	Mood swings, lack of focus
Decreased empathy	Digestive problems	Restlessness/irritability
More sick days	Sleep challenges	Extreme sensitivity
Lack of joy	Fatigue	Anxiety, rumination
Lack of purpose	Muscle tension/aches	Substance abuse
Self-doubt	Palpitations, high blood pressure	Depression, anger
Isolation	Chronic pain	Distraction
Difficulty concentrating	Decreased immune capacity	Hopelessness, numbness
Feeling overwhelmed	Clumsiness	Conflict

(Canadian Medical Association, 2020)

PROTECTIVE FACTORS

Protective factors are like personal protective equipment (PPE) that buffer us against burnout and compassion fatigue. While organizational and operational changes can serve as protective factors, this chapter focuses on three individual-level protective factors: compassion satisfaction, self-compassion, and social support.

COMPASSION SATISFACTION

Compassion satisfaction is the nourishment and fulfillment we feel from helping others (Sacco & Copel, 2017) and is associated with lower compassion fatigue and burnout

(Abou Hashish & Ghanem Atalla, 2023; Ruiz-Fernández et al., 2020), greater job satisfaction (Jialin et al., 2020), and improved patient safety (Ryu & Shim, 2022). Moments of compassion satisfaction can come from making a patient more comfortable, completing a successful procedure, feeling part of a team, or even saving a life. Compassion satisfaction works by counter-balancing the stress and demands of the job and thus mitigating fatigue and burnout.

Reflective practice is one strategy for fostering compassion satisfaction. This involves thinking about and sharing experiences with colleagues, expressing feelings, and sometimes gaining new perspectives. Regularly reflecting on our experiences can help us identify moments where we find meaning and satisfaction in our work, as well as providing an outlet to acknowledge and normalize the feelings of loss, sadness, frustration, and sometimes powerlessness that come with working in healthcare.

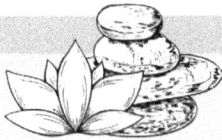

DESIGNING HARMONY EXERCISE 7.1

Reflective Practice Journal

Journaling allows you to reflect on challenges and rewards. Keep in mind that a single event may include both challenging and rewarding elements. Set up your journal pages accordingly (see Table 7.2).

Table 7.2 Reflective Practice Journal

Reward (Compassion Satisfaction)	Challenge
List a fulfilling or satisfying moment.	List a disappointing experience or struggle.
Reflect on the rewarding moment: • How did you feel about yourself? • What did you think or decide about yourself, your patient, or your coworkers? • What can you take away that will help you in the future?	Reflect on the struggle/challenge: • How did you feel about yourself? • What did you think or decide about yourself, your patient, or your coworkers? • Did you need any support or resources? • How can you get support in the future?

DEVELOPING SELF-COMPASSION

Self-compassion refers to how we relate to ourselves in moments in which we feel failure, inadequacy, or suffering. When we respond with a high level of self-compassion, we show ourselves kindness, understanding, and acceptance. When demonstrating low self-compassion, we may be self-critical and unforgiving (Neff, 2023). Self-compassion has three dimensions:

1. **Self-kindness vs. self-judgment:** Responding to ourselves with warmth and care rather than criticism

2. **Common humanity vs. isolation:** Recognizing our struggles are part of being human and feeling connected to others rather than feeling alone and isolated

3. **Mindfulness vs. overidentification:** Staying present and open to the full range of our experiences instead of being preoccupied with or defining ourselves by struggles or suffering

Fortunately, self-compassion is a skill that can be developed.

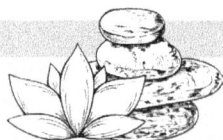

DESIGNING HARMONY EXERCISE 7.2

Developing Self-Compassion

Follow these steps to help develop self-compassion.

1. **Pretend you're a colleague:** Consider a difficult experience you had. Maybe you made a mistake or felt mistreated. Imagine a colleague had the same experience. Think about how you might respond to them. What words and tone would you use? Now think about the response you had to yourself. What is different? How would it feel to talk to yourself the way you might to a colleague?

2. **Add self-compassion to your reflective practice journal:** Return to your reflective practice journal. In your reflections, do you notice self-judgment or moments where you appear to feel alone or defined by your negative experiences? Write in the margins what you can say to yourself to show self-kindness, such as "you deserved grace that day," and common humanity, such as "anyone would have been overwhelmed."

(Adapted from self-compassion.org)

SOCIAL SUPPORT, MENTORSHIP, AND CAREER STAGES

Social support, particularly collegial support, has consistently been shown to reduce burnout and increase compassion satisfaction (Barr, 2017; Ruiz-Fernandez et al., 2021; Zhang et al., 2023). Additionally, professionals tend to experience stress and burnout differently as they move through their careers and utilize distinct coping tools across career stages, supporting the importance of mentorship and knowledge-sharing among colleagues with varying levels of experience. Reflect on your own career stage and how it may impact compassion satisfaction and burnout.

Consider reaching out to colleagues who can engage in reflective practice with you. Perhaps identify a "self-compassion buddy" to mutually support the development of self-compassion. What can you learn from both shared and distinct experiences?

Fostering practices in ourselves and our colleagues that promote protective factors can mitigate burnout and fatigue.

"The essence of healing emotional pain lies in listening to what hurts—in both knowing how to listen to oneself and being listened to by another."

–Miriam Greenspan, psychotherapist and author

LOSS AND MENTAL HEALTH

Grief and loss are expected components of working in healthcare due to the everyday experiences of patients' chronic suffering, disability, and death. When a patient dies during a shift, the healthcare worker's experience is referred to as *professional grief,* and the feelings that emerge in a clinical context are similar to grief experienced in a personal setting. The distinction, however, can be found in the absence of recognition from the world outside that the loss is impactful or significant. This *disenfranchised grief* has been connected to burnout (Lathrop, 2017), and avoidant responses of denial and emotional distancing are directly linked to burnout and low engagement (Zhang et al., 2023).

Healthcare systems are typically under-resourced for providing outlets for staff to engage with their emotional responses, and in fact, medical professionals are often trained to block emotions during crises. This expectation to suppress natural responses is often at odds with what is most beneficial for well-being. In professional settings, managing or controlling emotion is revered, and suppressing sadness, fear, or anger is preferred or even rewarded.

The increased consideration of emotions in the public discourse in recent years has not translated into knowledge about what to *do* with them. We are still so uncomfortable with emotions that even within the context of psychotherapy, healthcare professionals can struggle even to identify emotions, and merely naming feelings can be an achievement reached only after significant work.

Yet, listening to another's pain—simply being in the presence of pain—is difficult to filter. Our mirror neurons do not allow us to block experiencing the emotions of others, so we are left with regular exposure to pain in our healthcare roles without the tools to manage our own reactions.

Studies show that active emotional processing correlates with more positive outcomes, and when faced with adversity, positive psychological change—known as *posttraumatic growth*—can surface as a result of this processing. Posttraumatic growth may manifest as a stronger sense of self, new approach to life, shifts in spirituality, and increased openness to others, leading to more satisfying connections. Active and mindful experiencing of emotion has the potential to be transformative and catalyze personal and interpersonal growth. In contrast, compartmentalizing or suppressing emotional reactions can promote the inverse, such as poor physical and mental health, burnout, and fatigue.

Sometimes psychotherapy patients who have reached a significant moment of insight or recognized a deeply held emotion will ask, "So now what?" The answer is sometimes that nothing more is required—the mere act of turning an unknown feeling into an out-in-the-open verbalized thought means that a big step has been taken in emotional processing. When grief and loss are treated as emotions to be avoided, we create barriers to arriving at these critical moments of insight.

Miriam Greenspan's work on emotional alchemy (2003) provides one theory about how accepting and processing emotions directly and purposefully leads to new insights and understanding. *Emotional alchemy* is a call to recognize emotions, but instead of "thinking them away," it involves allowing oneself to be immersed in the feelings, as uncomfortable as that might be. It is less about moving through emotion and onto the next thing and more about settling in to learn more about the emotion and what it means for you. Trusting that the emotion has value for you will take you to a new level in learning about yourself and others. Ask the question, "Where will my grief take me?"

According to Greenspan, there are seven steps in turning grief into gratitude (see Table 7.3).

Table 7.3 Turning Grief Into Gratitude

1. Intention	Rather than wanting to be saved from feeling the difficult emotion, be curious to get to know the feeling better. Let yourself "be broken." Ask yourself, "What is my ultimate intention regarding this grief?"
2. Affirmation	This step calls for an "emotion-positive attitude" and asks that you befriend the emotion by approaching it as having something to teach you. In cognitive behavioral therapy, this is called *cognitive reframing*.
3. Bodily sensation	This step asks you to orient your attention to the physical sensations of grief. What do you notice in your body?
4. Contextualization	What story do you usually tell yourself about pain or suffering? Step 4 calls for widening that narrative and linking it to a larger cultural or social context to feel more connected in the shared human experience of pain.
5. The way of non-action	This step requires tolerating a feeling without immediately acting to stop or compartmentalize it. Mindfulness helps increase this capacity.
6. The way of action	Step 6 calls for letting yourself do things even if grief will accompany you. This could mean not isolating yourself from the grief.
7. Transformation: the way of surrender	This step calls for surrendering to the emotion to integrate the experience of grief into life going forward. Create new meaning through support or a creative outlet.

(Greenspan, 2003)

If the best route forward is to assess and experience the feelings you were trained to shut off, then moving forward requires time to turn your attention to these feelings. It also requires support from systemic resources, for "without a listener, the healing process is aborted" (Greenspan, 2003, p. 14). In a study of nursing staff working in COVID-19 wards, results suggested that reducing working hours, increasing ward rotations, and providing bereavement counseling would lead to a reduced experience of complicated grief (Rahmani et al., 2023).

DOPAMINE

Dopamine is a neurotransmitter getting much attention recently and is frequently cited in discussions related to addiction and attention deficit disorder, such as *Dopamine Nation* (Lembke, 2021) and *Dopamine for ADHD* (Russell, 2022). Connected to aspects as varied as sleep, movement, attention, mood, pleasure and reward, learning, and even lactation, dopamine is best thought of as a motivator for our internal reward systems. Chapter 2 discusses how dopamine might play a role in our experience of flow and immersive engagement in our daily lives. We now share strategies to actively manage your dopamine levels, which, when balanced, can be central to creating a sense of well-being and happiness. We seek dopamine throughout the day—often, this feels like a need for stimulation or distraction throughout the workday or in your life outside of work. Research tells us there are negative consequences to overzealous attempts to get dopamine boosts— our mental and physical health suffers from ingrained habits of turning to caffeine, sugar, and the ever-present scrolling on our phones to get through the day or to stave off boredom. We also know positive results are associated with choosing activities that lead to less immediate but longer-lasting boosts such as exercise, socializing, or engaging in activities we enjoy. "Dopamine menus" reduce our addiction to short bursts of dopamine while also strengthening habits that lead to long-lasting energy, resulting in better moods and higher engagement in daily life.

Everyone is susceptible to the negative impact of reliance on short-term rewards. When we are learning something new, dopamine helps us remember the good feelings we have and associate them so that we want to repeat that experience in the future. When dopamine levels are low, we are susceptible to losing our motivation to do what would bring us energy and joy. For instance, people with ADHD have dopamine in shorter supply (Grace, 2001) and thus often seek out activities with higher levels of reward or instant, short-term rewards. In fact, most people find that dopamine shortcuts work most reliably when first experienced, but over time, greater amounts are required to get the same result. These shortcuts to dopamine boosts are probably familiar to you in the form of social media scrolling, texting, or sugary foods. All these actions lead to immediate gratification and, you guessed it, dopamine surges. However, they do not help sustain ongoing energy levels, emotional regulation, or a sense of satisfaction or balance.

The dopamine menu (or "dopamenu") was initially popularized by Jessica McCabe (host of the popular YouTube channel "How to ADHD") and Eric Tivers (host of the podcast "ADHD Rewired") as a strategy for those struggling with focus and engagement. Dopamine menus have spread in popularity with professionals eager to increase engagement in their daily routine. Although yet to be studied as a tool for increasing wellness, research supports the underlying concept that physical exercise promotes dopamine's long-lasting release (Marques et al., 2021). Dopamine menus can be helpful in self-assessing responses to day-night shifts, seasonal shifts, and indoor working conditions. Because you create this menu in advance of when you need it, you are more likely to be intentional about the choices you make and end up with routines that will benefit you.

Consider a typical day when you cycle through a brief engagement period in a draining task, followed by frustration or exhaustion. Enter the quick chocolate bar to distract and boost your mood temporarily. Especially when experiencing burnout or lower energy levels, we do not tend to make well-thought-out choices, especially when rushed or in a hurry. The dopamine menu is an intentional approach to filling your day with things that are good for you and will lead to lower but sustained dopamine levels. Think of an intentional trip through the grocery store with an organized list and consider the opposite—a trip through the grocery store with no list while hungry! You are much more likely to check out with a cart full of quick calories to satisfy your hunger but less likely to have a cart full of ingredients for a healthy meal.

The first step is to create two lists. First, list all the activities you can rely on to elevate your engagement, focus, or mood. Second, list activities you tend to do when bored or resort to for a quick distraction (these typically make you feel worse and thus are best in moderation). Next, separate the first list of engaging activities into long versus short activities. Those that take more time or resources end up on the "main entrees," and the quick ones are your "appetizers." The second list—the distractions that drain your energy—will form your "desserts." One last step is to make a new list of small actions or activities to pair with less-enticing tasks to make them more engaging. These are your "sides." See Table 7.4 for examples of all four "menu items." Also, see the Appendix for ideas from established research about what increases dopamine and additional "dopamenu" ideas.

Remember that many of these activities, especially the appetizers, can be simple: drink water, cuddle with a pet, make a cup of tea, light a candle, and play music. The dessert list will likely be filled with the habits you want to break: Scrolling through social media provides a quick but short-term dopamine boost. Think of the dopamine menu as an active document—you may want to try only activities you already reliably go to for energy, or you may want to try out new ideas. Either way, the menu can be revised once you experience some success or failure. Try out a few versions and problem-solve if you cannot balance the categories. Dopamine menus are one way to achieve greater balance through increased focus, regulation, and engagement in an overstimulating world.

Table 7.4 Sample Dopamine Menu

Appetizers	Sides	Mains	Desserts
Make tea/coffee	Light a candle while doing paperwork	Long walk with a friend/ family member	TV series binge
Deep knee bends	Some caffeine	Workout	Social media scroll
Wordle	Listen to music	Dinner with friends	Real estate browsing
Hydrate	White noise	Do a puzzle	Sending reels
Quick walk	Use a heating pad	Cook a meal	Video games
Journal	Listen to an audiobook or podcast	Bake something	Sugary caffeine drink
Snack	Small sugary treat	Read a book in the tub	Social media posting
Tidy one small area	Stretching	Long conversation with a friend	Online shopping

A Systems Perspective on Healthcare Provider Mental Health

Healthcare provider mental health has far-reaching implications for the healthcare system, impacting the quality and perceptions of patient care and the high cost of turnover. The report by the National Academies of Sciences, Engineering, and Medicine from the Committee on the Future of Nursing 2020–2030 (2021) asserts that provider well-being is the responsibility of nurses, their employers, nursing schools, societies, professional organizations, and policymakers.

A Call for Action

Turnover and burnout lead to low morale within departments or teams and across systems, and the costs—for employee wellness, quality of patient care, and finances—are too high. Reduced quality and higher error rates can expose organizations to legal and reputational threats and further monetary burdens. Integrating mental health support into organizational culture will help to reduce the stigma that healthcare professionals face, which is a key barrier to their accessing mental health services.

Psychological Safety

Psychological safety (Edmondson, 1999; Tye, 2024) is the keystone of just culture and one that promotes well-being. It is the assurance that people can identify problems and errors, including their own, without fear of punishment, retribution, or humiliation. Its primary purpose is to eliminate patient safety incidents and encourage risk-taking innovation. Psychological safety is about the organization—emotional safety is about the individual. Investing in strategies to reduce overwork, improve job satisfaction, and build a climate of safety, recognition, and empowerment can improve well-being and enhance organizational performance. Chapters 5 and 6 explain the value of flexible scheduling and how to utilize it as one way to improve working conditions for employees.

Employee assistance programs provide confidential counseling and support for those experiencing burnout, anxiety, or depression and offer a compelling entry point that can reduce the barriers to accessing services. Contracting with mental health practices, facilities, or network groups to provide reduced fees or subsidized services can allow for a broader range of services, including longer-term care. Peer support programs can be invaluable in creating a sense of community and reducing feelings of isolation. Healthcare worker wellness impacts all aspects of the healthcare system and must be the concern of everyone touched by it.

BALANCE BREVITIES . . . ACTION STEPS

Here are four action steps to begin your journey:

1. Engage in reflective practice.
2. Identify a self-compassion "buddy."
3. Reflect on this: What can I learn about myself from my grief?
4. On your next work break, replace phone scrolling with a low-dopamine activity.

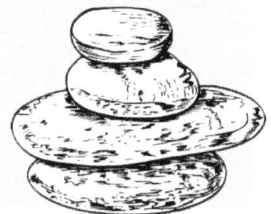

RESOURCES

MENTAL HEALTH

988 suicide and crisis line: https://988helpline.org/

Additional mental health resources, including links to wellness programs and free or low-cost services for healthcare professionals, can be found in the Appendix.

BURNOUT, COMPASSION FATIGUE, COMPASSION SATISFACTION, & SELF-COMPASSION

Self-compassion resources: https://self-compassion.org/

Self-compassion test: https://self-compassion.org/self-compassion-test/

REFERENCES

Abou Hashish, E. A., & Ghanem Atalla, A. D. (2023). The relationship between coping strategies, compassion satisfaction, and compassion fatigue during the COVID-19 pandemic. *SAGE Open Nursing, 9.* https://doi.org/10.1177/23779608231160463

Adams, R. E., Boscarino, J. A., & Figley, C. R. (2006). Compassion fatigue and psychological distress among social workers: A validation study. *American Journal of Orthopsychiatry, 76*(1), 103–108. https://doi.org/10.1037/0002-9432.76.1.103

American Nurses Association. (2023, May 19). *Nurse retention strategies: How to combat nurse turnover.* Nursing Resources Hub. https://www.nursingworld.org/content-hub/resources/nursing-leadership/nurse-retention-strategies/

American Nurses Foundation. (2025). *Pulse on the nation's nurses survey series: Annual assessment survey, November 2022.* https://www.nursingworld.org/practice-policy/work-environment/health-safety/disaster-preparedness/coronavirus/what-you-need-to-know/annual-survey--third-year/

Barr, P. (2017). Compassion fatigue and compassion satisfaction in neonatal intensive care unit nurses: Relationships with work stress and perceived social support. *Traumatology, 23*(2), 214–222. https://doi.org/10.1037/trm0000115

Canadian Medical Association. (2020, Dec. 8). *Compassion fatigue: Signs, symptoms, and how to cope.* https://www.cma.ca/physician-wellness-hub/content/compassion-fatigue-signs-symptoms-and-how-cope#:~:text=increased%20anxiety%2C%20sadness%2C%20anger%20and,nausea%2C%20upset%20stomach%20and%20dizziness

Cranage, K., & Foster, K. (2022). Mental health nurses' experience of challenging workplace situations: A qualitative descriptive study. *International Journal of Mental Health Nursing, 31*(3), 665–676. https://doi.org/10.1111/inm.12986

Edmondson, A. (1999). Psychological safety and learning behavior in work teams. *Administrative Science Quarterly, 44*(2), 350–383. https://doi.org/10.2307/2666999

Grace, A. A. (2001). Psychostimulant actions on dopamine and limbic system function: Relevance to the pathophysiology and treatment of ADHD. In F. M. Solanto, A. F. T. Arnsten, & F. X. Castellanos (Eds.), *Stimulant drugs and ADHD: Basic and clinical neuroscience* (pp. 134–157). Oxford University Press.

Greenspan, M. (2003). *Healing through the dark emotions: The wisdom of grief, fear, and despair.* Shambhala.

Hill, J. E., Harris, C., L., C. D., Boland, P., Doherty, A. J., Benedetto, V., Gita, B. E., & Clegg, A. J. (2022). The prevalence of mental health conditions in healthcare workers during and after a pandemic: Systematic review and meta-analysis. *Journal of Advanced Nursing, 78,* 1551–1573. https://doi.org/10.1111/jan.15175

Jialin, W., Okoli, C. T. C., He, H., Feng, F., Li, J., Zhuang, L., & Lin, M. (2020). Factors associated with compassion satisfaction, burnout, and secondary traumatic stress among Chinese nurses in tertiary hospitals: A cross-sectional study. *International Journal of Nursing Studies, 102.* https://doi.org/10.1016/j.ijnurstu.2019.103472

Lathrop, D. (2017). Disenfranchised grief and physician burnout. *Annals of Family Medicine, 15*(4), 375–378. https://doi.org/10.1370/afm.2074

Lembke, A. (2021). *Dopamine nation: Finding balance in the age of indulgence* [Unabridged]. Penguin Audio.

Letvak, S., Ruhm, C. J., & McCoy, T. (2012, May–June). Depression in hospital employed nurses. *Clinical Nurse Specialist, 26*(3), 177–182. https://www.doi.org/10.1097/NUR.0b013e3182503ef0

Maharaj, S., Lees, T., & Lal, S. (2019). Prevalence and risk factors of depression, anxiety, and stress in a cohort of Australian nurses. *International Journal of Environmentally Responsible Public Health, 16*(1), 61. https://doi.org/10.3390/ijerph16010061

Marques, A., Marconcin, P., Werneck, A. O., Ferrari, G., Gouveia, É. R., Kliegel, M., Peralta, M., & Ihle, A. (2021, June 23). Bidirectional association between physical activity and dopamine across adulthood: A systematic review. *Brain Sciences, 11*(7), 829. https://doi.org/10.3390/brainsci11070829

National Academies of Sciences, Engineering, and Medicine. (2021). *The future of nursing 2020–2030: Charting a path to achieve health equity.* National Academies Press. https://doi.org/10.17226/25982

Neff, K. D. (2023). Self-compassion: Theory, method, research, and intervention. *Annual Review of Psychology, 74,* 193–218. https://doi.org/10.1146/annurev-psych-032420-031047

Nigam, J. A., Barner, R. M., Cunningham, T. R., Swanson, N. G., & Chosewood, L. C. (2023, Nov. 3). *Vital signs:* Health worker–perceived working conditions and symptoms of poor mental health — Quality of worklife survey, United States, 2018–2022. *Morbidity and Mortality Weekly Report, 72*(44), 1197–1205. http://dx.doi.org/10.15585/mmwr.mm7244e1

Rahmani, F., Hosseinzadeh, M., & Gholizadeh, L. (2023). Complicated grief and related factors among nursing staff during the Covid-19 pandemic: A cross-sectional study. *BMC Psychiatry, 23*, 1–10. https://doi.org/10.1186/s12888-023-04562-w

Ruiz-Fernández, M. D., Ramos-Pichardo, J. D., Ibáñez-Masero, O., Cabrera-Troya, J., Carmona-Rega, M. I., & Ortega-Galán, Á. M. (2020). Compassion fatigue, burnout, compassion satisfaction and perceived stress in healthcare professionals during the COVID-19 health crisis in Spain. *Journal of Clinical Nursing, 29*(21–22), 4321–4330. https://doi.org/10.1111/jocn.15469

Ruiz-Fernández, M. D., Ramos-Pichardo, J. D., Ibañez-Masero, O., Sánchez-Ruiz, M. J., Fernández-Leyva, A., & Ortega-Galán, Á. M. (2021, November). Perceived health, perceived social support and professional quality of life in hospital emergency nurses. *International Emergency Nursing, 59*. https://doi.org/10.1016/j.ienj.2021.101079

Russell, M. (2022). *Dopamine for ADHD: Everything you need to know about brain stimulation with neurotransmitters such as dopamine to produce a motivation and carry out activities without any problems* [Unabridged]. Audible.

Ryu, I. S., & Shim, J. L. (2022). The relationship between compassion satisfaction and fatigue with shift nurses' patient safety-related activities. *Iran Journal of Public Health, 51*(12), 2724–2732. https://doi.org/10.18502/ijph.v51i12.11463

Sacco, T. L., & Copel, L. C. (2017). Compassion satisfaction: A concept analysis in nursing. *Nursing Forum, 53*(1), 76–83. https://doi.org/10.1111/nuf.12213

Tye, J. (2024). Creating a culture of emotional safety in healthcare. In S. Weinstein & D. Readinger (Eds.), *Healing healthcare: Evidence-based strategies to mend our broken system* (p. 39). Amplify Publishing Group.

World Health Organization. (2024, April 25). Protecting health and care workers' mental health and well-being: Technical consultation meeting. https://www.who.int/news/item/25-04-2024-202404_protecthw_mentalhealth#:~:text=%E2%80%9CParticularly%20 following%20the%20COVID%2D19,problems%20in%20our%20 workforce%2C%E2%80%9D%20stated

Zhang, J., Wang, X., Chen, O., Li, J., Li, Y., Chen, Y., Luo, Y., & Zhang, J. (2023, Nov. 13). Social support, empathy and compassion fatigue among clinical nurses: Structural equation modeling. *BMC Nursing, 22*(1), 425. https://doi.org/10.1186/s12912-023-01565-6

8

STRESS AND THE INFORMATION AGE

Sharon M. Weinstein, MS, RN, CRNI-R®, CVP, CSP, FAAN

In today's information-rich world, the challenge isn't accessing knowledge—it's navigating it.

Emerging technologies like virtual reality (VR), augmented reality (AR), holograms, and advanced simulations are transforming education. These tools immerse learners, turning abstract concepts into tangible experiences. VR allows users to enter historical events, AR enables virtual dissections, and holographic tutors offer lifelike interactions. While these innovations bridge the gap between overload and understanding, the key question remains: How do we balance engagement with effectiveness? This chapter explores managing stress and fatigue in the Information Age. Fatigue is a state of physical, mental, and/or emotional exhaustion.

THE OVERWHELM: THE STRESS CONNECTION AND ARTIFICIAL INTELLIGENCE

Overwork is a familiar challenge nurses face, driven by staffing shortages, increased patient acuity, and administrative burdens. The consequences of overwork are profound, affecting nurses' physical health, mental well-being, and job satisfaction. Prolonged periods of overwork can lead to various physical health issues for nurses. Chronic fatigue, musculoskeletal disorders, and cardiovascular problems are prevalent among those who work long hours without adequate rest. The physical toll of overwork is not limited to immediate health effects. Long-term exposure to high-stress environments can lead to chronic conditions such as hypertension, diabetes, and sleep disorders. These conditions affect the nurse's quality of life and ability to provide consistent, high-quality care. The physical strain of nursing, which often involves lifting patients, prolonged standing, and rapid response to emergencies, compounds the risk of musculoskeletal injuries (Weaver et al., 2024).

The rapid advancement of technology, constant connectivity, and artificial intelligence (AI) have transformed how we live and work. While the world is more connected than ever through smartphones, social media, and communication platforms, this connectivity has its drawbacks. It offers real-time communication and greater social interaction but also contributes to stress and fatigue. Constant notifications blur the line between work and personal life, leading to mental exhaustion, decision fatigue, and burnout. In this hyperconnected environment, the pressure to stay alert hampers recovery and well-being, creating significant challenges, such as:

- Work-life imbalance and the blurred boundary between work and personal life

- Sleep disruption from checking screens late into the night, interfering with sleep patterns
- Cognitive overload caused by the brain's inability to handle the constant flow of information we are exposed to daily

AI IN HEALTHCARE: THE GOOD, THE BAD, AND THE UGLY

In November 2022, Open AI launched ChatGPT, creating a new era in AI. Den Houter (2024) tells us that 93% of Fortune 500 chief human resource officers say their organization has implemented AI tools and technologies to improve business practices.

"Success comes to those who can skillfully blend artificial intelligence with authentic human insight."

–Lois B. Creamer, author of *More Business, Make MORE Money Speaking*

The release of ChatGPT in 2022 sparked a critical conversation on how new technology will reshape the labor market. AI tools like ChatGPT impact health, cognition, and performance by streamlining tasks and providing instant access to information. In healthcare and HR, ChatGPT automates administrative work, reducing time spent on repetitive tasks. It supports roles by allowing professionals to focus on complex, human-centered tasks. However, this may shift job requirements, creating demand for tech-savvy workers and reducing clerical positions. While it promises more accurate diagnoses and personalized treatment plans, healthcare professionals may also feel stress from overreliance on AI for decision-making, which can undermine their clinical judgment, leading to feelings of inadequacy. Excessive use of AI risks diminishing human skills, such as critical thinking, cognitive engagement, and communication, contributing to mental fatigue.

For patients, AI-driven technologies like predictive analytics and diagnostic tools can cause anxiety, especially when the results suggest higher risks or diseases, creating uncertainty. Finding a balance is crucial to ensure AI supports, rather than replaces, human capabilities and connections.

Does AI increase or decrease stress? Mark Herschberg answers that question for us in this quote:

"Tactically, [AI] can decrease stress by working as an unbiased and nonjudgmental partner who can help with brainstorming, editing, outlining, QA checks, and more. It can significantly improve overall efficiency, and learning to use it effectively can accelerate your career."

"Macroscale, AI also brings new stressors. On top of the stress stemming from any learning curve with new technology, many people rightly worry that if it automates enough tasks in their job, they need to adapt to a different set of responsibilities (change is scary) or could lose their job altogether (unemployment is more frightening)."

–Mark Herschberg, author, *The Career Toolkit,* and content creator, *The Brain Bump App*

LEVERAGING TECHNOLOGY TO ENHANCE EFFICIENCY

System issues that are the root cause of burnout must be fixed, such as work overload, understaffing, too many unnecessary bureaucratic tasks, and problems with the electronic medical record. Population health and well-being will improve only when a comprehensive multi-component strategy is implemented, including an evidence-based quality improvement approach that builds and sustains a culture of wellness.

We use multiple technologies within the work setting. Table 8.1 lists the most common technologies used in healthcare and what care providers need to know to use each effectively.

"As healthcare evolves, striking the right balance between staffing flexibility, patient safety, and technological integration is still a critical challenge for nurse leaders and healthcare administrators."

–Bob Dent, DNP, MBA, RN, NEA-BC, CENP, FACHE, FAAN, FAONL
Founder & Chief Executive Coach, DBD Coaching and Consulting

Table 8.1 AI Tools in Healthcare

Technology/Tool	Source	Need to Know
Electronic health records (EHRs)	Epic Systems, Cerner	Learn interoperability, data security
Telemedicine platforms	Doxy.me, Amwell	Privacy regulations (HIPAA) are crucial
Clinician decision support systems	Uptodate, IBM, Watson Health	Understanding integration of evidence-based information at the point of care
Wearable health technology	Fitbit, Apple Watch, Samsung Galaxy Watch	Interpret data for clinical decision-making
Remote patient monitoring	ResMed, Medtronic	Know how to integrate data into patient care plans
AI in diagnostics	Aidoc, Zebra	Focus on accuracy, limitations, bias
Mobile health apps	MyChart, Medscape	Know benefits, privacy concerns
Pharmacy management software	McKesson, Cerner	Understand drug interaction alarms
Radiology information systems	PACSHealth, Siemens	Know integration with EHRs and PACs
Virtual reality (VR)	Osso VR, Fundamental VR	Application for hands-on learning, skills development

Technology can significantly reduce workloads by streamlining administrative tasks, improving communication, and enhancing patient care. EHRs simplify documentation, ensuring quick access to patient information, reducing paperwork, and minimizing errors, allowing nurses to focus on care. Mobile health apps and telemedicine enable remote patient monitoring and timely interventions. Automated scheduling systems optimize shifts, balance workloads, and prevent burnout. By thoughtfully integrating these technologies, healthcare organizations can enhance efficiency, improve care, and alleviate the stress often experienced in demanding work environments.

- EHRs can improve care documentation and efficiency, but poorly designed systems can lead to excessive data entry and disrupt workflows. Healthcare organizations should involve providers in EHR design to meet clinical needs. Optimizing EHR systems, reducing redundant documentation, and providing training can save nurses time and reduce frustration.

- Telehealth and remote monitoring technologies have gained importance post-pandemic by reducing in-person visits and staff burden. They enable faster consultations, improve triage, and mitigate intensive care needs. However, successful implementation requires proper training, support, and clear guidelines to ensure nurses can effectively integrate these tools into existing workflows without feeling overwhelmed.

- Automation and AI in care delivery can revolutionize care by taking over routine tasks and allowing staff to focus on more complex aspects of patient care. AI algorithms can assist with medication management, patient monitoring, and predictive analytics, identifying patients at risk of deterioration and alerting nurses before a critical event occurs. This can reduce the cognitive load on nurses and enhance patient safety.

- VR and AR—now collectively called *extended reality,* or XR—allow us to reimagine education by simulating patient scenarios, creating opportunities for students to see the world as their patient sees it. According to Raderstorf (2024), XR offers immersive training experiences for healthcare students and professionals. These technologies function as modern simulation labs, enabling learners to practice complex procedures within a safe, controlled environment and better prepare the healthcare workforce.

While AI and automation offer significant benefits, ethical concerns like job displacement, data privacy, and dehumanization of care must be addressed. Nurses should be involved in discussions to ensure technology complements, not replaces, their work.

Establishing Healthy Digital Boundaries

"Innovation continually pushes the boundaries between the known and the unknown, offering immense potential to enhance the healthcare workforce. Progress is often the outcome when boundaries are tested. Recent advancements in healthcare, such as artificial intelligence (AI), telehealth, extended reality (XR), and wearable health devices, exemplify this progress."

—Tim Raderstorf, innovator, consultant

Information Overload and Its Impact on Mental Health

In Chapter 7, we address mental health in detail, but there are additional concerns with the effects of the Information Age. The rise of the internet and digital platforms has led to an explosion of information available at our fingertips. While this wealth of knowledge can be empowering, it also creates an environment of information overload. People are constantly bombarded with news, social media updates, and professional emails competing for their attention.

Social media platforms can exacerbate feelings of stress and anxiety. While they allow people to connect and share experiences, they can also foster feelings of inadequacy, comparison, and fear of missing out. Three of the most concerning aspects of social media consumption are:

- **Social comparison:** Constant exposure to idealized representations of others' lives on social media can lead to negative self-perception and stress.

- **Cyberbullying and harassment:** The anonymity provided by online platforms can also lead to cyberbullying, harassment, and online trolling, which can have serious consequences for mental health.

- **Fake news and information saturation:** The rapid spread of fake news and misinformation on digital platforms can increase stress and confusion. In a world where misinformation is quickly disseminated, people often feel unsure about what to trust, leading to paranoia and cognitive dissonance. This uncertainty can lead to mental fatigue, as individuals constantly try to discern the truth from the noise.

The mental health impact of social media—stemming from social comparison, cyberbullying, and misinformation—highlights a deeper concern about the potential physical risks of digital exposure. As we navigate constant stress and confusion online, we must also question the effects of prolonged exposure to electromagnetic fields (EMF) and radiofrequency (RF) radiation, which may exacerbate these issues.

FINDING BALANCE

EMF and RF Concerns

While not mainstream science or evidence-based at this time, EMFs are considered by some to be possible contributors to information overload, stress, and fatigue. Additionally, radiation from prolonged device exposure has been linked to potential risks like Alzheimer's, Parkinson's, and other neurodegenerative conditions (Berman & Sabol, 2016; World Health Organization ([WHO], 2002).

The potential for radiation exposure from Bluetooth devices, such as headsets and earbuds, arises from the low-level EMFs they emit. These devices emit RF energy and non-ionizing radiation (Environmental Health Trust, 2024). However, wireless devices, including earbuds, must meet specific absorption rate limits, which measure RF energy absorption by the body. Devices compliant with Federal Communications Commission (FCC) standards emit radiation levels that are considered safe. While the FCC (2020) and WHO (2025) state that current RF exposure levels from such devices are within safe limits, they continue to monitor ongoing research. Some experts and advocacy groups remain cautious about prolonged or close proximity use of wireless devices (FCC, 2020; Physicians for Safe Technology, n.d.).

The alleged physiological effects of EMFs include:

- **Chronic stress:** Continuous exposure to stressors, such as work demands, social media notifications, and information overload, can lead to chronic stress, which is linked to a range of physical health problems, including high blood pressure, heart disease, digestive issues, and a weakened immune system (Asamoah, 2023; Cho et al., 2022; Nathan & Shiloh, 2000).

- **Cortisol imbalance:** Chronic stress often leads to prolonged elevated cortisol levels, the stress hormone, which can disrupt normal bodily functions. High cortisol levels can interfere with sleep, digestion, and immune response, leading to various health issues (American Psychological Association, 2022; Zhou et al., 2024).

- **Other effects:** Exposure to EMF and RF fields from wireless devices may contribute to mental fatigue and loss of focus and interfere with melatonin production—thus disrupting sleep and making it harder for shift workers in particular to get restive sleep, which, among other things, aids in cellular repair (Khurana et al., 2010).

The alleged psychological effects of EMFs include:

- **Anxiety and depression:** The pressure to stay connected and the constant influx of information can lead to heightened levels of anxiety and depression.

- **Burnout:** The constant demand for attention and the expectation to be always available can lead to burnout, particularly in the workplace.

- **Cognitive decline:** Information overload and multitasking have been linked to decreased cognitive performance.

To minimize the potential negative effects, experts suggest limiting use of wired and wireless headsets or ear buds, alternating ears when they are used, and keeping handheld devices such as cell phones away from the body as much as possible.

COPING STRATEGIES AND SOLUTIONS

Overexposure to tech devices can lead to digital eye strain, causing headaches, blurred vision, and dry eyes. Tech neck, from poor posture, results in neck and shoulder pain. Excessive screen time disrupts circadian rhythms, leading to sleep disturbances. Constant notifications increase anxiety and stress, while prolonged inactivity harms physical health and reduces social interaction.. While research is ongoing, limiting screen time, using protective measures, and studying the long-term effects of tech device exposure are essential (Khurana et al., 2010; Mortazavi et al., 2023).

Awareness and moderate use are prudent strategies while research continues. Balancing use and breaks can help mitigate these effects. Just as electromagnetic interference from wireless technologies interferes with an airplane's or a hospital's equipment, it can interfere with our inner processes. We are electrochemical/electromagnetic creatures, as can be experienced when we hook up to an electroencephalogram or an electrocardiogram.

The rise of connectivity and AI has undeniably transformed how we live and work, bringing opportunities and challenges. While these technological advancements have enhanced communication, efficiency, and access to information, they have also introduced significant stressors that affect our mental and physical health. From constant digital connectivity and social media pressures to the demands of AI in the workplace and healthcare, we must remember that the impact on health is profound.

"In your thirst for knowledge, be sure not to drown in all the information."

–Anthony J. D'Angelo, author

Many individualized strategies recommended in the literature focus on the nurse adapting to stressors in their environment. Fiske and colleagues (2020) describe resilience as a complex personal characteristic that nurses may cultivate through trauma-informed strategies such as breathing exercises, expressing gratitude, and visual journaling. Hossain and Clatty (2021) describe the effectiveness of phone applications created to facilitate practical breathing exercises and mindfulness self-care activities. We should also continuously encourage an environment of self-care; fostering a culture of well-being as a nurse leader often means modeling self-care. See the Appendix to differentiate good stress (eustress) from bad stress; yes, there is a difference!

"Remember to empower yourself while you empower others. We as caregivers need to realize that we need to put on the oxygen mask first so we can help others."

–Alphonzo Baker, Sr., DNP, MSN, RN, CAPA, FASPAN
Immediate Past President, American Association of PeriAnesthesia Nurses

---

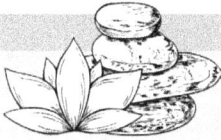

It's High Time for Digital Detox

Do your devices make your life easier or more challenging? Have you ever just wanted to be device-free? You have many "smart" devices and apps that facilitate your life's work, keep you on track and on time, turn on the lights and TV, and shut them down.

Is now the time for your digital detox?

Here are some ways to get "smart" about self-care:

- Set specific "offline" times: Designate certain hours, such as during meals or before bed, to disconnect from all devices and focus on personal well-being or relationships. You do it for family members, and you should do it for yourself.

- Create tech-free zones: Establish areas where devices are not allowed in your home or workspace, encouraging more mindful interactions and relaxation.

- Limit social media consumption: Allocate a specific amount of time each day for social media and stick to it, preventing excessive scrolling or comparison traps.

- Communicate availability expectations: Let family, friends, and colleagues know your preferred response times and boundaries for work-related communications outside business hours.

- Think about the communication tools you use and select one! Then, request your colleagues, family members, students, or clients to use that tool to communicate with you.

- Schedule breaks for yourself; even 15 minutes daily will make a massive difference in how you feel and perform.

- Add mindfulness to your routine while walking and eating.

- Make a gratitude list; think about people, places, and things that bring you joy.

Even though there is so much to do and so little time, take time for yourself and make being "smart" and balanced a part of your daily routine! You will thank yourself, and those around you will thank you, too. It's high time for a digital detox.

FINDING BALANCE

There's an App for That!

Table 8.2 lists 10 apps that support mindset, harmony, balance, and overall well-being, suitable for professionals and consumers.

Table 8.2 Mindfulness Apps

App	Purpose	Best For
Headspace	Mindfulness/meditation	New to meditation
Calm	Guided meditation, sleep stories, breathing	Sleep improvement/stress relief
Forest	Gamified time management	Procrastination
MyLife	Emotional check-ins/ personalized mindfulness	Tailored mental health support (does not replace professional therapy)
Strides	Goal-setting	Structured goal achievement
Daylio	Mood/activity tracking	Self-awareness/reflection
Insight Timer	Free meditation library	Cost-free wellness
Happify	Science-backed activities	Workplace stress
Reflectly	Positive thinking	Mental reset
Asana Rebel	Yoga, fitness/mindfulness combo	Fitness/mindfulness

HOW MUCH IS TOO MUCH?

How do you know when you have had enough? Are you overconnected to social media? Do you need to check your Facebook, Instagram, X, WhatsApp, TikTok, and LinkedIn accounts throughout the day? Can you divert your time and attention to activities that don't drain your balance? Can you use a program that posts for you once or twice weekly or twice daily to save time, energy, and exposure?

What is the impact of your social media use on your career, choices, and compliance? What can we do to tame our connectivity? How do we manage our time with the convenience of modern technology and respect for our health and our schedules? Many things can be done, but they all require commitment. It is like making a New Year's resolution—should it be a resolution or a commitment?

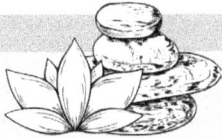

DESIGNING HARMONY EXERCISE 8.2

Aligning Yourself to Stay Connected and Safe

You can balance social media engagement and avoid becoming addicted. How you do that depends on your job, community, social circle, and need for connectivity. Can social media be a part of your work performance? The answer is yes if its use is work-related. To balance connectivity and safety, consider these principles:

1. Strengthen privacy settings.

2. Limit personal information sharing.

3. Be mindful of links and attachments.

4. Enable two-factor authentication.

5. Practice digital well-being.

BALANCE BREVITIES . . . ACTION STEPS

Limit exposure by:

- Digital detox: Take a break.

- Mindful consumption: Choose credible sources of info.

- Deep breathing and relaxation: Start now.

- Stay physically active.

- Establish boundaries, including "no-tech" times and zones.

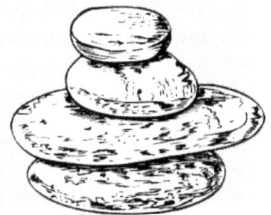

REFERENCES

American Psychological Association. (2022, Nov. 1). Media overload is hurting our mental health. Here are ways to manage headline stress. *Monitor on Psychology, 53*(8). https://www.apa.org/monitor/2022/11/strain-media-overload

Asamoah, T. (2023, Jan. 17). *Digital overload: Read this if your screen time is out of hand.* GoodRx. https://www.goodrx.com/health-topic/mental-health/what-is-digital-overload

Berman, S., & Sabol, W. (2016). Effects of electromagnetic fields on human health: A review of the literature. *Environmental Toxicology and Pharmacology, 47,* 13–21.

Cho, H., Sagherian, K., Scott, L. D., & Steege, L. M. (2022). Occupational fatigue, workload and nursing teamwork in hospital nurses. *Journal of Advanced Nursing, 78*(8), 2313–2326. https://doi.org/10.1111/jan.15246

Den Houter, K. (2024, Oct. 8). *AI in the workplace: Answering 3 big questions.* Gallup.com. https://www.gallup.com/workplace/651203/workplace-answering-big-questions.aspx?utm_source=gallup_brand&utm_medium=email&utm_campaign=ai_adoption_launch_us_3_november_11132024&utm_term=lead_generation&utm_content=continue_reading_here__textlink_2

Environmental Health Trust. (2024). *Do's and don'ts for safe technology.* https://ehtrust.org/wp-content/uploads/EHT-Dos-and-Donts-for-Safe-Tech-2-4.pdf

Federal Communications Commission. (2020, Nov. 4). *Wireless devices and health concerns.* https://www.fcc.gov/consumers/guides/wireless-devices-and-health-concerns

Fiske, E., Martin, S., & Luetkemeyer, J. (2020). Building nurses' resilience to trauma through contemplative practices. *Creative Nursing, 26*(4), e90–e96. https://www.doi.org/10.1891/CRNR-D-20-00054

Hossain, F., & Clatty, A. (2021). Self-care strategies in response to nurses' moral injury during COVID-19 pandemic. *Nursing Ethics, 28*(1), 23–32. https://www.doi.org/10.1177/0969733020961825

Khurana, V. G., Hardell, L., Everaert, J., Bortkiewicz, A., Carlberg, M., & Ahonen, M. (2010). Epidemiological evidence for a health risk from mobile phone base stations. *International Journal of Occupational and Environmental Health, 16*(3), 263–277. https://pubmed.ncbi.nlm.nih.gov/20662418/

Mortazavi, S. A., Haghani, M., Vafapour, H., Ghadimi-Moghadam, A., Yarbakhsh, H., Eslami, J., Yarbakhsh, R., Zarei, S., Rastegarian, N., Shams, S. F., Darvish, L., & Mohammadi, S. (2023). Should parents allow their children use smartphones and tablets? The issue of screen time for recreational activities. *Journal of Biomedical Physics and Engineering, 13*(6), 563–572. https://doi.org/10.31661/jbpe.v0i0.535

Nathan, C., & Shiloh, M. U. (2000). Reactive oxygen and nitrogen intermediates in the relationship between mammalian hosts and microbial pathogens. *Proceedings of the National Academy of Sciences, 97*(16), 8841–8848.

Physicians for Safe Technology. (n.d.). *Wi-Fi radiation health effects.* https://mdsafetech.org/wi-fi-effects/?utm_source=chatgpt.com

Raderstorf, T. (2024). Innovation and the healthcare workforce. In S. Weinstein & D. Readinger (Eds.), *Healing healthcare: Evidence-based strategies to mend our broken system* (p. 48). Amplify Publishing Group.

Weaver, S. H., Dimino, K., Fleming, K., Harvey, J., Manzella, M., O'Neill, P., Paliwal, M., Phillips, M., & Wurmser, T. A. (2024). Exploring sleep and fatigue of clinical nurses and administrative supervisors. *Nurse Leader, 22*(2), 203–210. https://doi.org/10.1016/j.mnl.2023.11.010

World Health Organization. (2002). *Establishing a dialogue on risks from electromagnetic fields* (pp. 5–62). https://www.who.int/publications/i/item/9241545712

World Health Organization. (2025). *The international EMF project.* https://www.who.int/initiatives/the-international-emf-project

Zhou, N., Qin, W., Zhang, J. J., Wang, Y., Wen, J. S., & Lim, Y. M. (2024). Epidemiological exploration of the impact of bluetooth headset usage on thyroid nodules using Shapley additive explanations method. *Scientific Reports, 14*(1), 14354. https://doi.org/10.1038/s41598-024-63653-0

V

PERSONAL AND PROFESSIONAL DEVELOPMENT

9

OPPORTUNITIES FOR GROWTH

Sharon M. Weinstein, MS, RN, CRNI-R®, CVP, CSP, FAAN

Now that you've reflected on and made strides toward harmonizing all aspects of your life, it's time to consider *who* that rebalanced you becomes in the workplace. Has your path led you to a forked road where "straight ahead" is no longer an option? Perhaps this is a personal choice because the organization has changed, and your skills no longer fit the new business focus. Or are you merely at a crossroads where you can continue on your present course but want to consider the options other directions offer? Regardless of what brought you to your present place, it may be time to take a deep breath and reflect on a new vision of what a career might mean for you.

ALIGNMENT AND ENGAGEMENT WITH LIFE'S PURPOSE

The first step to breaking free from a rut is acknowledging the need for change. Once you do, consider your direction: a new career, advancing in your current field, returning to a less stressful role you enjoyed, pursuing freelance or contract work, or taking a sabbatical. Reflect on how your life purpose and dreams align with your career goals. Explore meaningful activities with little or no financial compensation, such as art or missionary work. Use career-change exercises and resources like Quintessential Careers to guide your journey and make purposeful, fulfilling choices (https://www.livecareer.com/). Through career choice analysis, you can effectively plan and manage career change.

FINDING BALANCE

Employer Support for Advanced Degrees and Certifications

Supporting advanced degrees and certifications fosters growth, innovation, and expertise in the workforce, particularly in healthcare. Employers encouraging development through tuition reimbursement, flexible schedules, and study time demonstrate commitment, boosting morale, satisfaction, and loyalty. For professionals, advanced education enhances skills, career prospects, and earning potential while bringing cutting-edge knowledge and methodologies to their roles. Certifications add credibility and open pathways to leadership. Achieving these milestones requires significant investment, but organizations can ease the process with educational partnerships, mentorship programs, and clear career pathways. Pairing employees with mentors who've navigated similar journeys provides guidance and sets realistic expectations. By supporting education and growth, employers build a skilled, motivated workforce prepared to meet evolving demands, creating a win-win for professionals and organizations.

> "Innovation is the ability to see change as an opportunity, not a threat."
>
> —Steve Jobs, Apple co-founder

THE CORE VALUES INDEX

The Core Values Index (CVI) by Taylor Protocols measures innate preferences rather than learned behaviors. It uses a forced choice format comprised of only positive values; there are no negative disclosures. With a 97% repeat score reliability, it is the ideal tool to identify one's strengths. The CVI is an essential step in the quest for balance, putting you on a path to self-actualization (see Figure 9.1) and personal development.

Our core values are our innate self. They:

- Never change

- Exist from birth

- Arise from your intellect

- Are not learned behaviors

- Offer an essential view of who we are

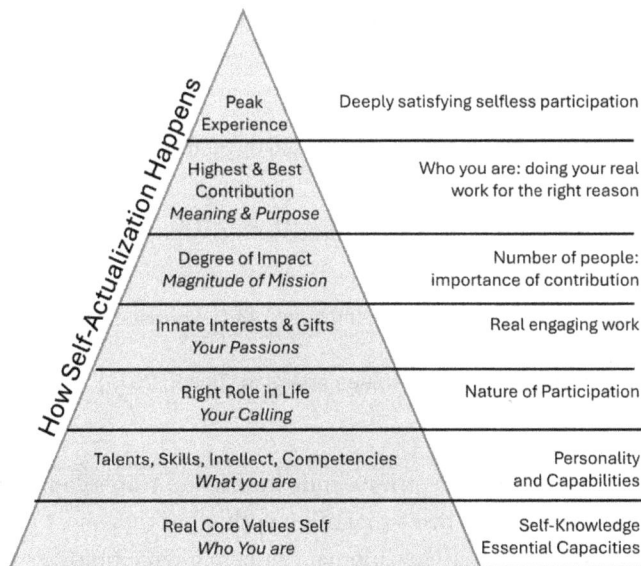

FIGURE 9.1 Taylor Protocols self-actualization pyramid (Taylor, 2012).

The CVI categorizes these core values (Taylor, 2012) into four primary types, often called "core values energies" (see Figure 9.2).

Builder	
Core Value:	Power – Focused on action and results
Catalyst:	Faith – Confidence in knowing what to do when
Team Contribution:	Driving outcomes through decisive action
Conflict Strategy:	May resort to intimidation
Learning Style:	"Decide and Do" – results oriented
Merchant	
Core Value:	Love – Focused on relationships
Catalyst:	Truth – Acceptance of things as they are
Team Contribution:	Building connections; inspiring shared vision
Conflict Strategy:	May be manipulative
Learning Style:	"Talk and Listen" – Engage in storytelling
Banker	
Core Value:	Knowledge – Focused on facts and data
Catalyst:	Justice – Ensures fairness, accountability
Team Contribution:	Ensuring wise use of resources
Conflict Strategy:	May respond with aloof judgment
Learning Style:	"Read and Analyze" – Prefers data
Innovator	
Core Value:	Wisdom – Focused on problem-solving
Catalyst:	Compassion – Empathetic
Team Contribution:	Creativity, ideation
Conflict Strategy:	May interrogate or intimidate
Learning Style:	"Access and Solve" – Prefers discovery process

FIGURE 9.2 Core values energies (Taylor, 2012).

By understanding these core motivations, individuals and teams can leverage their natural strengths and find roles or tasks that align with what they most value. The CVI is commonly used in organizational development to help align employees with tasks that match their core values, enhancing engagement, productivity, and overall job satisfaction.

You can access a complimentary CVI assessment via the QR code in Figure 9.3 or by going to https://members.taylorprotocols.com/Tools/CVIGift. aspx?GiftHash=19c9dd39-762c-1037-9eee-a667101c5d7d.

FIGURE 9.3   CVI QR code.

PROFESSIONAL COACHING

Professional coaching empowers you to be your best, feel your best, and do your best in your business, personal life, and career search. By starting with your life's purpose and identifying what is essential, your goals are set, and you can begin the implementation process. Coaching works because you have an objective partner in the process; your coach helps you to reach the competitive edge that sets you apart from others and establishes you in your field. Your coach enhances your ability to solve your problems with action-oriented practical strategies, an accountability system that keeps you motivated, a fresh perspective to challenge your limiting beliefs, and support when you need it most. From platform skills to improved performance, a coach may lead the way.

THINK DIFFERENTLY

In an earlier chapter, you learned about design thinking and the 4Ws approach. Have you ever been told to think outside of the box? How did that make you feel? Were your ideas not good enough? Has fear held you back and kept you inside the box? Fear is a powerful force that sometimes makes that box feel safe from thoughts like:

- What if it doesn't work?

- What will people think?

These fears can freeze us in our tracks. But here's the truth: Fear is not the enemy. It's a sign that you're on the brink of an outside-of-the-box idea!

"Thinking outside the box" is a metaphor for thinking differently or beyond the limits of the box-like structure.

My journey began in a box, where I was told to learn to type because I would never amount to anything. But I didn't let that define me. I rolled up my sleeves, learned to type or use a keyboard, and went further. I learned to think differently (Readinger & Weinstein, 2022), challenge authority, and be the change I wanted to see. I learned to type using a manual typewriter with blank keys and typed 150 words per minute.

These lessons have been my guiding light, showing me the power of thinking differently and asking the right questions to solve the correct problems at the right time.

Imagine your mind as a flashlight. When you shine it in one direction, you see what's in front of you, but everything else remains dark. Now, imagine swiveling that flashlight and illuminating other things. This is thinking differently: moving the flashlight and exploring the shadows that may have held you inside the box, stagnating your career!

Thinking differently begins with questioning conventional wisdom and exploring uncharted territories. It requires a willingness to take risks, an openness to new ideas, and the resilience to learn from failures. By doing so, you position yourself as a forward-thinker and a problem-solver, attributes highly valued in any industry.

When you dare to think differently, you differentiate yourself from your peers. Employers and leaders notice those who bring fresh perspectives and innovative solutions. This distinction can lead to greater visibility, new opportunities, and accelerated career growth. For instance, by identifying a gap in the market and proposing a novel solution, you can spearhead projects that showcase your leadership potential and strategic thinking. Thinking differently fosters a growth mindset essential for personal and professional development. It encourages continuous learning and adaptability, ensuring relevance in an ever-evolving job market. The courage to think differently can inspire and motivate teams in leadership roles. Leaders who champion unconventional ideas and support calculated risks create an environment where creativity and innovation thrive.

ASKING "WHAT IF . . . ?": USING THE 4WS ON YOUR CAREER PATHWAY

How can you use the concept of thinking differently to grow in your career? Gather diverse groups from within and beyond your network. Using the 4Ws technique, asking "What if" questions can help you gain new perspectives on your career and identify potential paths for change.

STEP 1

What is the current situation? Listen to and engage with others who know your work so that you can assess the current state of your career. Get their feedback and clarify where you want to be in your short- and long-term career.

STEP 2

Reframe the challenge by asking "What if?" and begin brainstorming.

Explore career possibilities. Imagine multiple career paths that align with your interests and skills:

- Consider job roles or opportunities you could explore.

- Develop a clear vision of where you want to be. What if everything goes according to plan? What does success look like for you?

Use What if? statements to generate innovative ideas. For example, instead of "How can I get a promotion?" ask:

- What if I pursued a different role within my current organization?

- What if I sought additional training or education?

- What if I explored opportunities in a different industry?

What if? encourages you to think creatively about potential career paths and the skills needed. It's about envisioning various possibilities and identifying growth opportunities through new roles, upskilling, or cross-departmental projects.

STEP 3

Next, prioritize "What wows?"—what is doable, and what investments of time, talent, and dollars are needed. Is it upskilling, taking credentialing courses, or returning to school?

Identify the opportunities or actions that can have the most significant positive impact on your career. These are the game-changers. This stage is about pinpointing what will create the most value for the individual and the organization. What wows? focuses on leveraging unique strengths and finding roles or projects that have the potential to make a substantial impact, accelerating career growth.

STEP 4

The last step— "What works?"—takes the best ideas from steps 1, 2, and 3 and uses small-scale prototypes to gather feedback, improve a potential solution, and wash, rinse, and repeat. Small-scale prototypes allow you to test and refine ideas before implementing them on a larger scale:

- Start with simple, low-cost prototypes such as sketches, paper models, or digital wire frames.

- Create multiple iterations of the prototype, each time incorporating feedback and improving the design.

- Test, gather feedback, and refine:

  - Launch pilot programs to test the refined prototype in a real-world setting with a larger audience.

  - Monitor performance and make further adjustments.

  - Once validated, implement the solution on a full scale, ensuring it meets the needs of the broader audience.

What works? is about taking actionable steps toward career development. It involves creating a structured plan, leveraging feedback, and adapting to change. This phase ensures that career aspirations translate into tangible achievements through deliberate and consistent effort.

This can reshape our career trajectory. This human-centered approach includes those for whom one is designing and puts them at the center of the design.

"Ask the right questions, and the answers will always reveal themselves."

–Oprah Winfrey

The mindset to re-imagine what's possible is a powerful catalyst for career acceleration. It sets you apart, fosters continuous growth, and positions you as an asset and leader. Embrace this mindset, and you'll find yourself on a fast track toward success and fulfillment in your professional journey.

Thinking differently and solving the right problems at the right time is about asking the right questions, overcoming fears, and persistently shining your flashlight into the dark corners of possibility. The path beyond the box starts with a single step: the courage to think differently. So, let's roll up our sleeves, move that flashlight, and see what we can illuminate together.

WATCH OUT FOR THE STUMBLING BLOCKS

THE AMYGDALA

The *amygdala* is a small, almond-shaped structure located deep within the brain's temporal lobe and is a critical limbic system component. It plays a crucial role in processing emotions, particularly fear and pleasure. The amygdala evaluates sensory information and triggers emotional responses, influencing behavior and decision-making. It also helps form emotional memories, allowing individuals to remember experiences associated with strong feelings. By interacting with other brain regions, the amygdala significantly contributes to survival mechanisms, helping to assess threats and initiate appropriate reactions, such as fight-or-flight responses.

When tensions rise, the amygdala is triggered, and the hippocampus reminds us that a lack of response equates to, "I am unworthy; my gut says to jump in, but I simply cannot do it." The mind can play tricks on us, so you have to "train your brain" to step in, step up, and ask for what you want. See Chapter 4 for strategies to grow self-regulation, develop grit, and other ways to manage stress.

IMPOSTER SYNDROME

A persistent feeling of self-doubt despite evident success is a common barrier to career advancement. This is called *imposter syndrome.* As professionals advance in their careers, they may feel inadequate or question their qualifications, even when their achievements demonstrate competence. This can lead to reluctance to seek promotions, hesitation to share ideas, or avoidance of challenging roles, which may stall career growth.

To combat imposter syndrome, practice self-reflection by acknowledging past successes and skills that have led to your current role. Mentorship helps to provide external validation and guidance, often revealing that feelings of self-doubt are common, even among seasoned professionals. Setting small, achievable goals can help build confidence. By recognizing that growth usually involves discomfort and self-doubt, you can reframe imposter syndrome as a natural part of career development and find the confidence to pursue advancement assertively. See the Appendix for more about avoiding imposter syndrome.

"I have written 11 books, but each time I think, 'Uh oh, they're going to find out now. I've run a game on everybody, and they'll find me out.'"
–Maya Angelou, American poet, author, and activist

REWIRE OR PREFERMENT?

Ask yourself the following nine questions. Then, examine your responses and identify what you must do to be balanced. For example, if the items on your bucket list are out of reach, you need to change something in your schedule to allow you to have those experiences.

1. Identify the people, places, and activities that give you joy today.

2. What is your vision for your future?

3. List five things on your bucket list.

4. Do you plan to work beyond age 60?

5. Do you plan to stay in the same kind of role long term?

6. What will change for you if you change careers?

7. What will change for you if you stop working?

8. Do you currently do volunteer work or serve on a board?

9. Are you and your life partner on the same page?

Why are you here today? Why are you reading this book? Consider two well-known figures—Charles Schulz and Ernest Hemingway—to evoke contrasting perspectives on aging and life experiences. Schulz maintained his creativity and influence, suggesting that "over the hill" does not mean slowing down; it can mean gaining momentum. The more careful Hemingway, known for his deliberate writing style, seemed to adopt a more thoughtful, measured outlook in his later years (Castro, n.d., 2016; Hendrickson, 2011).

"Your core values provide the compass that keeps you moving in the right direction."

—Susan David, PhD, author of *Emotional Agility*

What's your situation? Have you been in your present position for a year, two years, or more? Are you in a dead-end position that seems to lack a future? Do you hate your boss, or are you the boss?

Is it time for you to rewire or choose your preferred option? I have done it several times. Growing up with parents who told me to learn to type because I would never amount to anything, I was challenged at an early age to be the best. As the middle of five kids, I did not have the "middle child syndrome," but I did have the "caught in the middle syndrome," and it was not fun! So, I started at an early age to identify ways to better myself, learn and do more, achieve great heights, and start all over again.

I entered nursing school because I liked people, got a scholarship from the Philadelphia public schools, and had a safe place to live. I loved patient care. I often thought that there were patients who could not recover without my presence every shift. I worked harder and smarter than many of my classmates, and I was a good student, albeit impatient. I always anticipated the next step, the next part of the obstacle course, the next challenge.

As I think back, I realize that part of my wish to reinvent myself stemmed from a lack of self-esteem and an awareness that others were brighter and kinder than I was and that they came from what seemed to be (at least on the outside) loving families. So, part of the rewiring process involved giving myself a new look and career. I was able to shine beyond my wildest dreams and worked hard at it.

People rewire and reinvent themselves for different reasons. For some, it's the sudden realization that they're not happy or fulfilled, commonly called a midlife crisis. On the other hand, the reinventors prefer "finding themselves," particularly when they're not in the mood to admit that they're flat-out bored and need a change. Some of you may have kids who are still finding themselves, or you may be that person yourself.

Consider the following as you rewire yourself:

- Keep your options open. Don't turn down opportunities just because they are outside of the parameters of what you have thought to be your job title or place in life.

- Cross-pollinate. Take your knowledge, skills, and abilities from one field to another. Step outside your comfort zone.

- Follow your heart's desire and your dream. Your heart is a wise barometer of what you need to be doing with your life. Think from the heart as well as the mind when you evaluate opportunities.

The traditional concept of retirement is evolving as individuals seek greater fulfillment and flexibility in their later years. Retirement has long been associated with the end of a career and the beginning of a leisurely, passive phase of life. However, as life spans increase and attitudes toward work and leisure shift, many individuals are rethinking this traditional path. Preferment (Weinstein, 2024), a concept that prioritizes personal fulfillment and flexible engagement in meaningful activities, is emerging as a compelling alternative.

Preferment is a proactive approach to career transition that emphasizes doing what we want, with whom we wish to, and when we want. By shifting the focus from winding down to pursuing passions and meaningful activities, preferment offers a more fulfilling and personalized alternative to conventional retirement.

Preferment is about designing a life that aligns with one's passions, interests, and values, regardless of age. It involves choosing activities and engagements that bring joy and satisfaction, often blending work, leisure, and personal development elements. Critical aspects of preferment include:

- **Autonomy:** The freedom to decide how, when, and with whom to engage in various activities

- **Purpose:** Pursuing activities that provide a sense of meaning and contribution

- **Flexibility:** Adapting one's schedule and commitments to fit personal preferences and lifestyle

- **Continuous growth:** Embracing lifelong learning and personal development

The benefits of preferment include:

1. **Enhanced well-being:**

    a. Mental and physical health: Engaging in preferred activities can boost mental health by reducing stress and increasing happiness. Staying active and engaged can also benefit physical health.

    b. Life satisfaction: Preferment encourages focusing on what truly matters to the individual, leading to higher overall life satisfaction.

2. **Social connections:**

    a. Meaningful relationships: Individuals can cultivate deeper, more meaningful relationships by choosing with whom to spend time.

    b. Community engagement: Preferment often involves community activities, fostering a sense of belonging and social support.

3. **Continued contribution:**

    a. Utilizing skills and experience: Many preferment activities leverage the skills and experience accumulated over a lifetime, allowing for continued contribution and relevance.

    b. Mentorship opportunities: Experienced professionals can mentor younger generations, providing guidance and sharing knowledge.

4. **Financial flexibility:** Preferment may include diverse income streams such as part-time work, consulting, or entrepreneurial ventures, offering financial flexibility without the constraints of full-time employment.

WHEN OPPORTUNITY KNOCKS, ANSWER

We are in a never-ending state of change. We are constantly growing and evolving, and it is impossible to remain the same person you are today, even if you want to. Think about your career and the number of times that you have reinvented yourself.

"Once you find your purpose, you can radically change your life for the better and impact the lives of your family and community in the years to come."

–Anna Dermenchyan, PhD, RN, interim Chief Quality Officer, UCLA Department of Medicine

---

When you began your career, you likely envisioned yourself as a clinician or educator, focused on the next step. Over time, you specialized, honed your skills, and became an expert (Benner, 2013; Eustace, 2020). You may have taken on leadership roles within your organization, joined professional groups, or even started a local chapter or national position.

"Human beings have an inalienable right to invent themselves."
–Germaine Greer, author

BALANCE BREVITIES . . . ACTION STEPS

Here are four action steps to identify and create growth opportunities:

1. Conduct self-assessment.
2. Seek feedback and mentorship.
3. Pursue professional development.
4. Network and build relationships.

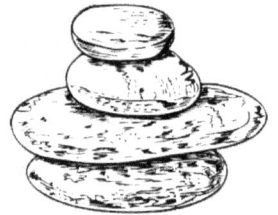

REFERENCES

Benner, P. (2013). *Nursing theories: From novice to expert.* Current Nursing. http://currentnursing.com/nursing_theory/Patricia_Benner_From_Novice_to_Expert.html

Castro, T. (n.d.). *When we all wanted to be Hemingway.* https://tonycastro.substack.com/p/when-we-all-wanted-to-be-hemingway

Castro, T. (2016). Looking for Hemingway: Spain, the bullfights, and a final rite of passage. Lyons Press.

Eustace, R. (2020, Aug. 21). *From novice to expert.* Nursology. https://nursology.net/2024/08/06/from-novice-to-expert-overnight-the-hidden-toll-of-rapid-advancement-on-nursing-burnout/

Hendrickson, P. (2011). Hemingway's boat: Everything he loved in life, and lost, 1934–1961. Alfred A. Knopf.

Readinger, D., and Weinstein, S. (2022). *Think differently: 18 strategies to fix broken thinking.* SMW Group.

Taylor, L. E. (2012). *The core values handbook* (2nd ed.). Elliot Bay Publishing.

Weinstein, S. M. (2024, Aug. 5). From retirement to preferment: Crafting your next chapter. *American Nurse Journal.* https://www.myamericannurse.com/from-retirement-to-preferment-crafting-your-next-chapter/

"I seldom end up where I wanted to go, but almost always
where I need to be."

–Douglas Adams, writer and humorist

10

YOUR FUTURE . . .
YOUR LIFE

Sharon M. Weinstein, MS, RN, CRNI-R®, CVP, CSP, FAAN

Whether you call it balance, integration, harmony, or something else, you must find the right formula that works for you. Celebrate your successes, and don't dwell on your failures. Life is a process, and so is striving for balance. A universal law that is the basis of all economic and personal well-being describes how to put the law to work for you, increase your effectiveness, and experience a more abundant life.

BLENDING A FULFILLING LIFE WITH A MEANINGFUL ONE

We all assume many roles in life—in the family, the workplace, the physical community, and the professional community. Each role enables us to express a different dimension of our being. It is these separate roles that need to be balanced in our lives. For example, if you are professionally successful, your life requires balance, but your family complains that you do not spend enough time with them. If your career is soaring again, your lifestyle needs balance, but your health is challenged. Finally, if you are addicted to a favorite TV show but have no time to clean your closets or the garage, your life needs balance.

"Gather only what you need; travel lightly, and keep moving forward. The journey will be more joyful with less baggage."
–Deborah Haggerty, writer

Table 10.1 compares the concepts of harmony and balance; it illustrates how they each contribute to overall well-being differently.

Table 10.1 Harmony vs. Balance

Aspect	Harmony	Balance
Definition	A state where different elements coexist peacefully and complement each other	A condition where different aspects are equal or proportionate, often requiring adjustments
Focus	Emphasis on synergy and integration among various components	Focus on equal time, energy, and resource distribution among competing demands

Approach	More fluid and adaptable, allowing for changes based on circumstances and emotions	More structured, often requiring a conscious effort to maintain equilibrium
Outcome	Results in a fulfilling and enriching experience, promoting well-being and contentment	Results in stability, ensuring that no single aspect dominates over others
Perspective	Encourages embracing differences and finding ways to work together harmoniously	Encourages systematic planning to allocate time and resources fairly

Blending a fulfilling life with a meaningful one requires a focus on purpose, connection, and well-being. In a demanding field like healthcare, professionals often strive to make an impact while balancing personal and professional growth. Here's how you can harmonize fulfillment and meaning:

- **Align with purpose:** Knowing your "why" provides resilience and drives meaning in daily tasks.

- **Nurture connections:** Engage with your team and foster trust and collaboration. Meaning grows when you feel connected to others working toward shared goals, while personal fulfillment thrives on these rich, supportive relationships.

- **Prioritize self-care and growth:** Remember that lesson from the first edition of *B Is for Balance:* "Self-care is *not* selfish."

Balancing these elements enables you to find joy and purpose while contributing to a healthier world.

"The Joy in the Journey . . . This Is Nursing! As I think of my nursing career, I now realize how blessed I am—for the journey, the experience, and the people who have impacted my life and helped me find my purpose."

–Benjamin Joel Breboneria, DNS, MA, MSN, RN, CNE, NEA-BC, Global Health Leader, Commissioner/NLN, Academic Program Director

---

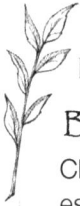

Best Practices for Work-Life Harmony

Claiming your life in the pursuit of work-life harmony involves setting clear priorities, establishing boundaries, and practicing self-compassion. Best practices in support of this journey include:

- **Define your values and priorities:** Identify what truly matters to you across work and personal domains. Reflect on the areas that bring you the most fulfillment, whether it's career growth, family time, personal development, or health. Use these priorities to guide decisions, helping you focus on what aligns with your values.

- **Establish firm boundaries:** Set boundaries that protect your time and energy. Communicate these boundaries openly with colleagues and loved ones, whether reserving specific hours for family or limiting work-related notifications outside of business hours. Boundaries ensure that each part of life gets the attention it deserves without unnecessary overlap.

- **Practice self-compassion:** Achieving harmony takes patience. Recognize that balance looks different at each life stage and is subject to change. Practice self-compassion by accepting imperfections and giving yourself grace when things don't go as planned. This mindset helps maintain **resilience and prevents burnout.**

Claiming your life is about taking control with intentional choices, which fosters harmony and enriches all facets of your life.

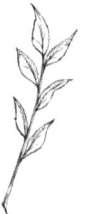

BALANCING PROFESSIONAL GROWTH WITH PERSONAL RESPONSIBILITIES

In today's fast-paced work environment, advancing professionally often demands time, energy, and focus that can strain personal life. The key to achieving this balance is setting clear priorities, establishing boundaries, and practicing intentional growth.

By aligning growth goals with your values, you can make career choices that enhance—not compete with—personal responsibilities. This alignment makes it easier to navigate complex choices, such as deciding whether a new project, role, or course truly supports your overarching goals.

Setting boundaries is equally crucial. Protecting family, health, and leisure time helps prevent burnout and ensures engagement at home and work.

Finally, approach growth intentionally. Rather than striving for every opportunity, focus on meaningful, strategic steps with the most significant impact. With clear priorities and boundaries, professionals can foster growth while honoring personal commitments.

WHAT ARE YOU THINKING?

Your mindset is everything: It will make or break you. Mindset is a set of assumptions, methods, or notions held by one or more people that drive behavior, choices, and outcomes. Strive to integrate your life's physical, emotional, mental, and spiritual aspects. Establish respectful, cooperative relationships with your family, friends, community, and the environment. Make the internal dialogue with yourself positive as you pursue your goals.

"We like to think of our champions and idols as superheroes born different from us. We don't like to think of them as relatively ordinary people who made themselves extraordinary."
–Carol S. Dweck, psychologist, writer

CHANGE YOUR MIND AND CHANGE YOUR LIFE

We realize that change happens, and we must be prepared to evaluate, value, and implement the change. Change is inevitable. Changing your mind reshapes your perspective, unlocking new possibilities. By embracing a growth mindset, you empower yourself to adapt, overcome limitations, and create a life aligned with your highest potential.

Focus on changing your mind and changing your life. First, you must understand change to be open to the process and realize the effects.

BECOMING THE BEST VERSION OF YOU

You've heard the term, and now, how do you do it?

How do you become the best version of *you*?

Becoming the best version of yourself involves embracing personal growth, self-compassion, and purpose-driven action. Start by clarifying your values and setting meaningful goals aligned with them. This alignment guides your decisions, making it easier to prioritize what truly matters.

Next, commit to lifelong learning. Cultivate a growth mindset by seeking new skills, knowledge, and experiences that challenge and expand your capabilities. Personal development flourishes when you actively explore areas of improvement but remember to celebrate progress along the way.

Practicing self-compassion is also essential. Recognize that setbacks are part of growth, not failures. Embrace them as learning opportunities rather than obstacles, and be kind to yourself.

Finally, lead a purpose-driven life. Invest your energy in pursuits that align with your passions and positively impact others. By focusing on both personal growth and contributing to the world around you, you'll become the best, most fulfilled version of yourself.

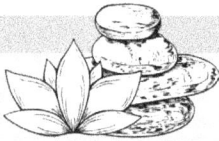

Limiting Beliefs

Overcoming limiting beliefs requires a mix of self-awareness, intentional action, and resilience. These beliefs often develop from past experiences, fears, or societal expectations, and they can significantly hold you back if not addressed. Here's a guide to breaking free:

- **Identify and acknowledge limiting beliefs:** Start by recognizing the specific thoughts that keep you from reaching your potential. Common limiting beliefs might include thoughts like "I'm not good enough," "I don't deserve success," or "Failure is too risky." Write down these beliefs to make them tangible and challenge their origins.

- **Reframe your mindset:** Once you've identified limiting beliefs, work on replacing them with empowering ones. For example, instead of thinking "I'll never be a good leader," reframe it as "I am learning to be a better leader every day."

- **Take action to build confidence:** Start small. Each time you take a step outside your comfort zone, you prove to yourself that you're capable of more than you previously believed. Action is the antidote to fear; even small achievements can create momentum. Celebrate these wins, no matter how small, as they gradually build the self-confidence needed to overcome self-imposed limitations.

- **Commit to continuous growth:** Adopt a growth mindset that embraces learning and adaptability. By viewing challenges as opportunities to grow, you're less likely to feel trapped by limiting beliefs.

Overcoming limiting beliefs is a process, not a one-time fix. With time and consistency, you'll replace doubt with confidence and start reaching new heights in both your career and personal life.

> "The future of a nation lies in the hands of its youth and their ability to share the generations to come."
>
> –Nelson Mandela

GENERATIONAL CONCERNS

The healthcare workforce is becoming increasingly multi-generational, with Traditionalists, Baby Boomers, Gen X, Millennials, Gen Z, and yes, Gen Alpha, all contributing to the workforce and organizational success (see Figure 10.1). While this diversity brings valuable perspectives, it challenges communication, technology adoption, and workplace dynamics. Understanding generational differences is essential for fostering a collaborative environment, optimizing productivity, and ensuring quality care. (Pearce, 2024). For example, "pay" and "location" are top-five job considerations among younger team members. To get by, side hustles have become more common, and more than half of these side hustles are within the healthcare space (Hines, 2024). Leaders must embrace these differences to create inclusive, effective, and adaptable teams in an evolving healthcare landscape.

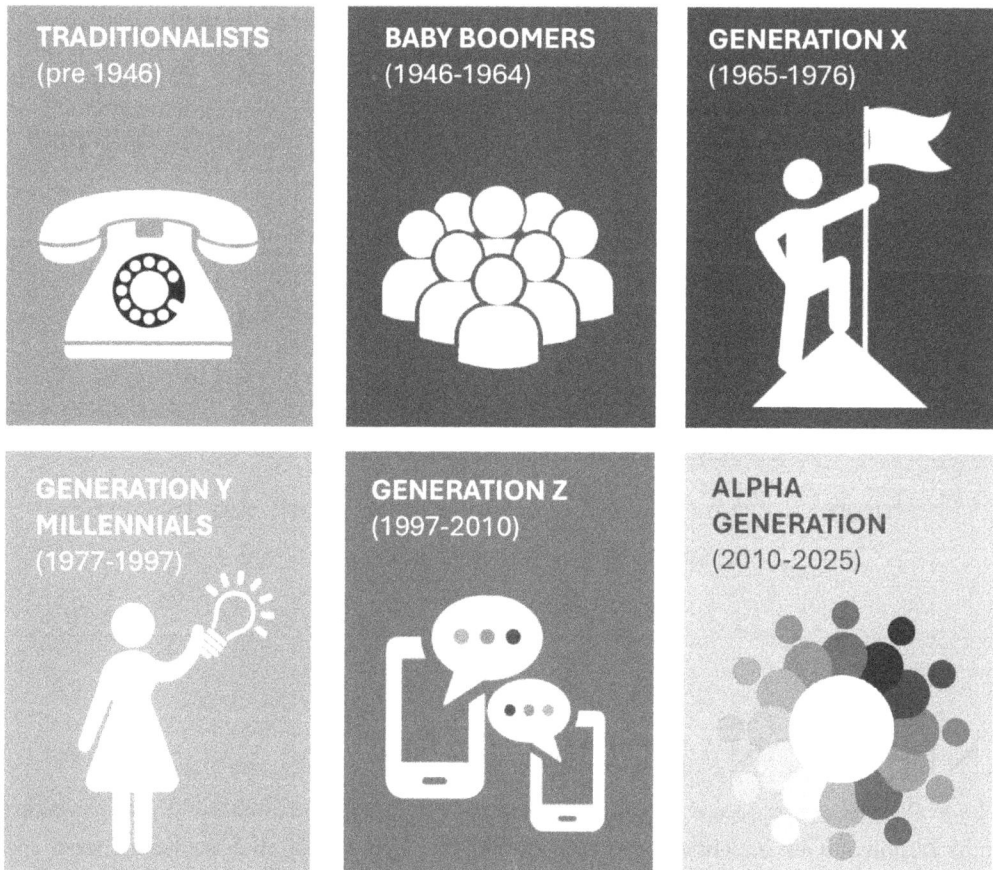

FIGURE 10.1 Generations in the workplace.

Each generation brings its own set of values, life stages, communication preferences, and priorities. Managers and leaders who can effectively understand, communicate with, motivate, train, and retain employees across four or five generations are highly sought after in every industry, from technology and healthcare to finance and retail. This ability is a critical skill for leaders navigating today's diverse workforce.

TRADITIONALISTS

An increasing number of seasoned workers are postponing retirement and returning to the workforce. Traditionally, this group grew up with clear rules, discipline, and a focus on goals. While not every Traditionalist's experience was the same, many were raised to be seen but not heard and to focus on hard work and responsibility. As Traditionalist nurses return to the workforce, their wealth of experience and wisdom becomes invaluable in mentoring and guiding new graduates. By sharing their knowledge, they help bridge the gap between academic learning and real-world practice, fostering a supportive and knowledgeable environment for new nurses to thrive:

- **What makes them tick:** Traditionalists value structure and may feel uncomfortable with technology, but they often have younger family members who help them adapt. They are driven by loyalty and seek recognition for their years of experience. Positive feedback and performance reviews help reinforce their sense of value.

- **How to motivate and reward them:** Traditionalists are often motivated by formal recognition, such as job titles and compensation, and appreciate acknowledgment of their loyalty and hard work. To keep them engaged, provide opportunities for face-to-face communication and create mentorship programs that allow them to share their wisdom.

BABY BOOMERS

Baby Boomers are known for their hard work, ambition, and resilience. They are not risk-averse and often thrive in leadership roles:

- **What makes them tick:** Boomers are highly ambitious and value self-worth and career success. Work/life harmony can be challenging for them, as they are accustomed to a more traditional work structure. They enjoy having insight into career development opportunities and are motivated by promotions, career advancement, and financial rewards.

- **How to motivate and reward them:** Boomers appreciate status symbols, such as promotions, and view performance reviews as necessary but uncomfortable. They prefer flexible working conditions, added benefits, and opportunities to remain in the workforce longer, sometimes even opting for *preferment*—continuing their work as long as they choose, without an early retirement push.

- **How to ensure they aren't left behind:** Boomers prefer group decision-making and tend to excel in collaborative environments. They thrive under flexible management styles and are used to shaping workplace dynamics. Communication with Boomers is often more formal and guarded, and they value the opportunity to contribute their expertise in leadership positions. To ensure they are not left behind, create a supportive work environment where their experience is recognized and appreciated. Many of them have already sought preferment—remaining on the job as long as they like and not seeking an early retirement. Their preference drives their productivity (Weinstein, 2024).

By understanding these generational groups' unique needs and preferences, managers can foster a more cohesive and productive work environment for all employees.

GEN X: WORK TO LIVE, NOT LIVE TO WORK

- **What makes them tick:** Gen Xers, often raised in dual-income or single-parent households, were the original latchkey kids, returning to empty homes after school. Many witnessed economic instability, like layoffs and downsizing, which shaped their view of job loyalty and security. They value change and prefer informal work environments, and they may change jobs frequently to seek greater freedom and satisfaction.

- **How to motivate and reward them:** Gen X values work-life balance and flexibility. They are direct, collaborative, and responsive to feedback. Allow them space to manage their time and pursue their interests while meeting professional goals.

- **How to ensure they aren't left behind:** Leaders should offer Gen X autonomy and opportunities to contribute ideas and strategies. As the first generation to transition from analog to digital, they adapt well to new technology, and leveraging these skills can enhance their productivity.

GEN Y (MILLENNIALS): THE ECHOBOOMERS

- **What makes them tick:** Millennials, raised with Baby Boomer parents, are digital natives who can't imagine life without the internet. They often look for new opportunities to advance and improve their skills, with job tenures typically ranging from six to 18 months. Known for their opportunistic mindset, they may learn from you but then move on to better opportunities.

- **How to motivate and retain them:** Millennials crave feedback and career development. They need clear communication and alignment between job descriptions, expectations, and reality. To retain them, growth opportunities and regular mentoring should be offered.

- **How to ensure they aren't left behind:** Provide challenging projects, foster their professional development, and offer mentoring opportunities to keep Millennials engaged. They thrive when their work is meaningful, and they expect to be continuously challenged and inspired.

GEN Z: THE DIGITAL NATIVES

- **What makes them tick:** Gen Z values salary but cares more about the meaningfulness of their work. They are split between the desire for high pay and fulfilling, interesting tasks. As the most racially and ethnically diverse generation, they value diversity and inclusivity in the workplace.

- **How to attract them:** To attract Gen Z, focus on inclusivity, sustainability, and social responsibility. Use gender-neutral language in job postings and demonstrate a commitment to addressing societal issues like climate change and inequality.

- **How to ensure they aren't left behind:** Give Gen Z the tech tools they love and encourage face-to-face communication for feedback. They appreciate autonomy in managing their projects and want to contribute ideas. Provide a work environment that allows them to grow and feel heard.

GENERATION ALPHA: THE DIGITAL INNOVATORS

- **What makes them tick:** Generation Alpha, the first fully digital generation, is accustomed to seamless technology integration. They value innovation, immediacy, and adaptability. Purpose-driven work and ethical alignment with employers are also important to them.

- **How to attract them:** Organizations should highlight their commitment to digital integration, flexibility, and social responsibility. Emphasize sustainability and innovation in your brand, showing a commitment to ethical leadership and global challenges.

- **How to ensure they aren't left behind:** Offer personalized learning and mentoring programs tailored to their digital skills. Foster a flexible work environment that values continuous growth, allowing Generation Alpha to contribute meaningfully while aligning with their passion for innovation and social impact.

While Generation Alpha may not yet be old enough to pursue a healthcare career, they are certainly at an age where they can begin to evaluate whether this type of work aligns with their values and fits into their future lives. Including Generation Alpha in this book is important, as it encourages early reflection on career choices and how they can integrate personal values with professional aspirations in healthcare.

KEY TAKEAWAYS

- **Diverse perspectives:** Each generation offers unique skills and experiences that enrich patient care and problem-solving.

- **Technology adaptation:** Younger generations are more tech-savvy, but older workers may require additional support with new systems.

- **Communication styles:** Generational communication preferences (e.g., digital vs. face-to-face) can impact teamwork and effectiveness.

- **Mentorship:** Cross-generational mentoring helps bridge knowledge gaps and fosters mutual respect.

- **Flexibility:** Offering flexible schedules or work arrangements supports retention and satisfaction across all generations.

THE POWER OF A MULTIGENERATIONAL WORKFORCE

A workforce that embraces input from diverse generations encourages innovation, creativity, and collaboration. Each generation brings its strengths, from Gen X's adaptability to Millennials' drive for purpose to Gen Z's tech-savviness to Gen Alpha's forward-thinking mindset. By recognizing and valuing these differences, organizations can build stronger, more inclusive teams better equipped to thrive in a rapidly changing world.

CREATING YOUR FUTURE

"It's time for nurses to step into their power—saying NO to disease-care and YES to healthy, proactive healthcare models. Imagine nurses being encouraged to think outside the box and disrupt the status quo. Nurses have the potential to create, develop, and implement new models of care focused on wellness and disease prevention that are both affordable and accessible."

–Dina Readinger, founder of Diagnostic Design Thinking and co-author of *Think Differently* and *Healing Healthcare*

FIND YOUR PASSION

Passion is what turns the ordinary into the extraordinary. Take time to reflect on what excites you—list things you love doing, people you admire, and places you want to go. When you visualize your passions, you're more likely to achieve them.

To uncover your true passion, explore activities that energize and engage you. Try different fields, hobbies, or roles that align with your values. Ask yourself, "What impact do I want to make?" Set flexible goals that adapt to new opportunities and changing interests, and see them as stepping stones to your future success.

A BLUEPRINT FOR SUCCESS

In healthcare, our work is more than a job—it's our purpose. Success comes from staying focused on your goals. Understanding who you are is a key part of that focus. Discover your true calling, especially in nursing, and let that guide your path.

"As a nurse, there are many opportunities for growth and career shifts. You'll find a pathway that aligns with your talents and interests. With the demand for healthcare professionals high and opportunities plentiful, leap. Choose an educational program that equips you with the skills to succeed in the future of healthcare."
–Jacqueline Dunbar-Jacob, PhD, RN, FAAN, Dean Emeritus, Distinguished Service Professor of Nursing, University of Pittsburgh

---

BALANCE BREVITIES . . . ACTION STEPS

Here are four action steps for creating a harmonious future in your life:

1. Set clear goals.
2. Prioritize well-being.
3. Cultivate relationships.
4. Establish boundaries.

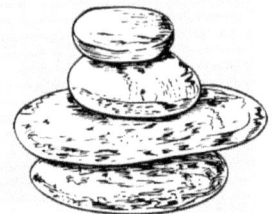

REFERENCES

Hines, M. (2024, Feb. 20). *The Vivian healthcare workforce report.* https://hire.vivian.com/blog/vivian-healthcare-workforce-report-2024

Pearce, N. (2024, April 4). Leading the 6-generation workforce. *Harvard Business Review.* https://hbr.org/2024/04/leading-the-6-generation-workforce

Weinstein, S. M. (2024, Aug. 5). From retirement to preferment: Crafting your next chapter. *American Nurse.* https://www.myamericannurse.com/from-retirement-to-preferment-crafting-your-next-chapter/

APPENDIX

CHAPTER 1

ALTERNATE VALUES CARD SORTING STRATEGIES & PROCEDURES

Multi-step values card sorts allow individuals to compare values across different points in time. For example, if you're early in your career, you might first sort cards based on current values, then sort again to reflect future aspirations. Comparing these sorts can reveal patterns, differences, and actionable steps for achieving desired transitions. Multi-sorter sorts, on the other hand, compare individual responses to others or organizational values, highlighting the fit between personal and professional environments.

APPLICATIONS OF MULTI-STEP SORTS

1. Now and later:

    a. Compare present values with those anticipated in 5–10 years.

    b. Transition insights: school to work, work to retirement, or energy focus versus true values

2. Person-organization fit:

    a. Align personal values with organizational culture or job-specific values.

    b. Team leaders can use sort results for role assignments.

    c. During hiring, card sorts identify critical values and skills for candidate evaluation.

3. Multi-sorter applications:

    a. Team-building: Visualize and reflect on collective values.

    b. Gain external perspective: Have peers rank your demonstrated versus internal values.

EXPANDING CARD SORT OPTIONS

- Create custom cards tailored to specific contexts, such as therapy or personal growth. For example, couples might create cards representing needed support and compare rankings to identify gaps.

- Use non-verbal cards featuring images or abstract designs to explore emotions or ideas. These are particularly effective in therapy, team dynamics, or with children and adolescents.

Individuals and teams can deepen self-awareness, improve relationships, and align values with goals or environments by customizing and applying card sorts.

HEROES AND ROLE MODELS

Table A.1 Heroes and Role Models Reflection

Step	Key Reflection Questions	Example
Identify a Role Model	Who do you admire, and what value do they embody?	Example: A peer who consistently shows empathy and kindness.
	When did you first observe this value in them?	Example: During a stressful project, they stayed calm and supportive.
	What actions or behaviors demonstrate this value?	Example: They actively listen, show patience, and offer thoughtful feedback.
	How did witnessing these actions make you feel?	Example: Inspired and motivated to be more patient with others.
	Which behaviors or characteristics would you like to emulate?	Example: Listening without interrupting and offering constructive support.
	What strengths or abilities did they demonstrate?	Example: Strong communication skills and emotional intelligence.
	What can you learn from their example?	Example: The power of calm leadership during high-pressure situations.

continues

Table A.1 Heroes and Role Models Reflection (cont.)

Step	Key Reflection Questions	Example
Reflect on Yourself	What in your behavior reflects this role model's influence?	Example: I try to stay calm in challenging conversations.
	What strengths, skills, or passions align with this value?	Example: I'm naturally empathetic but need to improve active listening.
	How can you apply those strengths?	Example: Practicing mindfulness to stay grounded in conversations.
	What challenges or skill gaps make it difficult to live this value?	Example: I sometimes interrupt when I'm anxious or in a rush.
	What knowledge or experience do you need to improve?	Example: Learning conflict resolution techniques to manage tension.
Overcome Obstacles	What obstacles are in your way?	Example: Time constraints and feeling overwhelmed.
	What can you control or influence?	Example: I can create a plan to manage my schedule better.
	Who can help you overcome these challenges?	Example: A mentor or coach who excels in conflict resolution.
	How can you ask for help from this person or resource?	Example: Schedule a meeting to ask for guidance and practical tips.

CHAPTER 2

MINDFULNESS: BEGINNER'S MIND EXERCISES

Choose a moment in your day to view your surroundings from a child's perspective. For example, as you walk to your car, notice the world as if it is new. Observe the color and sound of a bird, and feel the texture of the pavement underfoot. Below are additional exercises to cultivate Beginner's Mind:

Flip your expectations: When confronted with a situation in which you assume you know the outcome, take a moment to notice your assumptions. What if you approached this task as if everything you believed was not true? This exercise encourages you to question your beliefs and broaden your perspective.

Slow down: Physically slow your pace as you move through your day so your mind can fully notice the world around you. This isn't just about moving slowly; it's about permitting yourself to be present in each moment.

Notice the fortune-teller in you: Throughout your day, you may predict what will happen—perhaps assuming your supervisor will be irritated or that a co-worker will forget something. These predictions can color your experiences and actions. Instead, practice waiting and observing what happens without assumptions.

Be curious: Practice asking more straightforward questions like "Why do you do it that way?" or "Can you explain more about that?" By approaching conversations with genuine curiosity rather than assumptions, you open yourself to new perspectives and deeper understanding.

Imagine this is the only time: Approach tasks as if you will only complete them once. Viewing each action as unique brings a heightened sense of mindfulness and intention.

Let go of being the expert: Embrace a Beginner's Mind by letting go of the need to be right or the desire to always have the answers. Approach tasks, conversations, and experiences with an open mind, as if you are starting from scratch.

Adapted from Patrick Buggy, "How to Cultivate Beginner's Mind for a Fresh Perspective" (2020): https://mindfulambition.net/beginners-mind/)

Mindful Eating: Practicing Beginner's Mind

Mindful eating is another way to practice Beginner's Mind. It involves holding present-moment awareness and paying attention to your eating experience. Choose any piece of food to practice with; for this example, let's use a raisin. To prepare for this exercise, turn off all distractions—phones, computers, televisions, etc. Approach the raisin with the curiosity of a child who has never seen one before or is from a place where raisins do not exist.

Examine the raisin's physical traits—its texture, wrinkles, weight, and feel. Is it sticky or squishy? Notice the fine details on its skin. Please take a moment to smell the raisin and breathe in its odor. Close your eyes if it helps. Listen to the raisin—does it make a sound if you shake it or press it?

Notice your body's sensations as you bring the raisin to your mouth and anticipate tasting it. Consider how it feels to hold the raisin before biting it. As you chew, notice the taste—sweet, slightly sour, or bitter. How does it feel in your mouth? What sensations do you experience when you bite into it, chew it, and swallow it?

Finally, commend yourself for trying this exercise. This practice helps you become more mindful of the present moment and cultivate a deeper awareness of your surroundings and experiences.

Adapted from Mindfulness for Beginners *(Kabat-Zinn, 2012)*

CHAPTER 3

RECOGNIZING A BREAKING POINT WITH NURSE FATIGUE

SIGNS OF NURSE FATIGUE

- **Chronic physical exhaustion:** Constant tiredness despite rest

- **Emotional burnout:** Irritability, anxiety, or detachment from patients and colleagues

- **Decreased job performance:** Errors or reduced care quality from mental and physical fatigue

- **Physical symptoms:** Persistent headaches, muscle pain, or gastrointestinal issues

- **Neglecting self-care:** Skipping breaks, vacations, or feeling guilty about rest

Fatigue compromises personal well-being and patient safety—recognizing these signs is critical to preventing burnout.

FIVE ACTION STEPS TO PREVENT NURSE FATIGUE FROM REACHING A BREAKING POINT

1. **Foster a supportive work culture**

   Organizational action: Build an environment where breaks, vacations, and seeking help are encouraged. Promote open communication about workloads and well-being.

   Individual action: Nurses should prioritize self-care and feel empowered to communicate their needs. Speaking up when overwhelmed is crucial for personal and patient safety.

2. **Prioritize rest and recovery**

   Organizational action: Implement shift structures for adequate breaks and time off. Flexible scheduling supports nurses' recovery needs.

   Individual action: Nurses must commit to taking breaks, leaving on time, and using vacation days without guilt to restore energy.

3. Promote wellness and mental health support

Organizational action: Provide access to counseling, Employee Assistance Programs (EAPs), and mental health training to identify burnout early.

Individual action: Nurses should engage in wellness programs, use stress-reduction techniques, and seek professional support.

4. Manage workload realistically

Organizational action: Adjust staffing to prevent overburdening nurses. Use technology or support staff for administrative tasks.

Individual action: Nurses should set boundaries, delegate tasks, and prioritize essential duties to avoid burnout.

5. Encourage peer support and collaboration

Organizational action: Foster team collaboration through peer check-ins, mentorship programs, and sharing coping strategies.

Individual action: Nurses should rely on colleagues for emotional and practical support, building strong, supportive teams.

By fostering well-being and open communication, organizations and nurses can reduce fatigue, ensuring safer care and healthier work environments.

CHAPTER 4

ALIGNMENT: HNHN AND AACN ESSENTIALS

The Healthy Nurse, Healthy Nation (HNHN) initiative by the American Nurses Association (ANA) directly supports the American Association of Colleges of Nursing (AACN) *Essentials* by promoting nurses' physical, mental, and emotional well-being. This alignment ensures nurses are prepared to deliver high-quality care, improving healthcare outcomes.

1. PATIENT-CENTERED CARE

- HNHN alignment:

  - *Personal health and wellness:* By focusing on nurses' well-being, HNHN ensures nurses have the physical and mental energy to provide empathetic, patient-centered care. Healthier nurses engage more effectively with patients.

  - *Empathy and communication:* Stress management and wellness initiatives enhance nurses' ability to communicate with compassion and maintain emotional connections with patients.

2. TEAMWORK AND COLLABORATION

- HNHN alignment:

  - *Workplace wellness programs:* HNHN promotes workplace initiatives that improve teamwork, fostering supportive environments where nurses collaborate effectively.

  - *Healthy work environment:* A focus on reducing burnout and stress through wellness programs enhances collaboration and team cohesion, leading to better patient outcomes.

3. EVIDENCE-BASED PRACTICE

- HNHN alignment:

  - *Promoting research and education:* HNHN encourages nurses to engage with health and wellness research, translating these findings into evidence-based practices in patient care.

- *Health promotion and prevention:* Nurses model healthy behaviors through wellness programs, promoting preventive care strategies for patients and themselves.

4. QUALITY IMPROVEMENT

- HNHN alignment:

  - *Continuous improvement in health practices:* Nurses engaged in personal wellness are better positioned to contribute to quality improvement initiatives within clinical settings.

  - *Safe practice environments:* By advocating for safer workplaces and healthier practices, HNHN helps reduce workplace injuries, an essential component of quality improvement.

5. SAFETY

- HNHN alignment:

  - *Reducing occupational hazards:* HNHN addresses critical safety issues like needlestick injuries, ergonomic risks, and chemical exposures, directly improving workplace safety.

  - *Stress and fatigue management:* Managing nurse fatigue and stress through wellness programs enhances patient safety by reducing errors.

6. INFORMATICS

- HNHN alignment:

  - *Health informatics tools:* HNHN leverages technology to monitor nurses' wellness metrics, providing actionable data for improving workforce health policies.

  - *Technology in wellness programs:* Tools like fitness apps and virtual mental health resources help nurses manage their well-being, integrating informatics into daily practice.

CONCLUSION

The Healthy Nurse, Healthy Nation initiative aligns seamlessly with the AACN *Essentials* by prioritizing nurse wellness, fostering safer work environments, and ensuring high-quality patient care. By addressing nurses' holistic health, organizations empower nurses to meet professional competencies while enhancing the overall safety and effectiveness of healthcare delivery.

ALIGNING AACN ESSENTIALS WITH WORK/LIFE INTEGRATION

The AACN *Essentials* highlight key competencies for nursing practice, including patient-centered care, teamwork, and safety. However, achieving these competencies requires balancing professional demands with personal well-being.

CHALLENGES TO WORK/LIFE INTEGRATION

Nurses face unique challenges:

- Long, irregular shifts and physically demanding work
- Emotional stress, leading to burnout and job dissatisfaction

STRATEGIES FOR INTEGRATION

1. **Organizational support:** Develop policies promoting work/life balance, such as leadership-driven, family-friendly initiatives and wellness programs.

2. **Flexible scheduling:** Offer shift flexibility, job-sharing, or part-time roles to allow nurses control over their schedules, improving job satisfaction.

3. **Mental health resources:** Provide counseling, stress management programs, and peer support groups to help nurses cope with emotional demands.

4. **Professional development:** Encourage education and growth opportunities that align with AACN competencies, keeping nurses engaged while enhancing skills.

Aligning the AACN *Essentials* with strategies for work/life integration fosters sustainable nursing careers. By prioritizing nurse well-being, healthcare organizations can improve retention, reduce burnout, and ensure high-quality care. Nurse leaders must champion these strategies to create environments where nurses thrive professionally and personally.

CHAPTER 5

TIPS FOR MANDATORY OVERTIME

Mandatory overtime is a reality in many industries, particularly healthcare, retail, and manufacturing. While it can feel overwhelming, you can manage the extra hours without sacrificing your well-being or work-life balance with the right strategies. Here are three tips to help you navigate mandatory overtime effectively:

1. **Prioritize self-care:** Working extra hours can quickly lead to burnout if you don't care for yourself. Make sure to get enough sleep, eat nutritious meals, and stay hydrated. Scheduling regular breaks during your shifts can also help you recharge and maintain focus. Physical activity, such as stretching or short walks, can relieve tension and prevent fatigue.

2. **Set boundaries:** While mandatory overtime is often unavoidable, it's essential to communicate your limits. If overtime is becoming excessive, discuss possible alternatives with your supervisor, such as adjusting your shift schedule or reducing hours later. Having clear boundaries helps prevent burnout and shows your commitment to your health and productivity.

3. **Stay organized:** Planning is vital to managing extra work hours. Use a planner or digital calendar to schedule your work and personal commitments. By staying organized, you can ensure you're using your time efficiently, leaving space for rest and personal activities.

By following these tips, you can maintain your well-being and stay productive, even during mandatory overtime.

And, when all else fails, recall these two quotes from the first edition of *B Is for Balance*, published by Sigma in 2012:

- NO is a complete sentence!
- Self-Care is NOT selfish!

CHAPTER 6

Managing Fatigue, Night Shifts, and Shift Work Disorder

Working night shifts or irregular hours can lead to significant fatigue and even shift work disorder (SWD), affecting those with rotating or overnight schedules. SWD disrupts the body's natural circadian rhythms, leading to sleep disturbances, difficulty staying awake during work hours, and exhaustion during off-hours. The relationship between fatigue, night shifts, and SWD is complex. While night shifts can cause sleep deprivation, the lack of proper rest and recovery increases the risk of developing SWD, negatively impacting physical health, mental well-being, and job performance.

To manage the challenges of night shifts and combat fatigue, here are five tips for success:

1. **Avoid energy drinks:** While they offer a temporary boost, energy drinks can disrupt sleep and increase dehydration. Opt for water or herbal teas instead.

2. **Prioritize sleep:** Establish a consistent sleep routine. Try to sleep in a dark, quiet environment to simulate nighttime rest.

3. **Take strategic breaks:** Schedule breaks throughout your shift to recharge, stretch, and move your body.

4. **Support wellness around the clock:** Ensure your workplace has a wellness program available 24/7 to provide staff with wellness resources and guidance during all shifts.

5. **Practice healthy eating:** Choose light, nutritious meals that provide sustained energy and avoid heavy, greasy foods that can make you sluggish.

Implementing these strategies can reduce fatigue and prevent shift work disorder, improving overall health and performance during night shifts.

CHAPTER 7

SUICIDAL IDEATION: SIGNS & SYMPTOMS, DO'S AND DON'TS FOR INTERVENTION

Table A.2 Signs & Symptoms of Suicidal Ideation (SI)

Indicators of Suicidal Thinking and Risk			
Emptiness	Talking about death, wanting to die	Guilt, shame	Hopelessness, despair
Feeling trapped	Feeling like a burden to others	Believing they have no options	Extreme sadness
Giving possessions away	After intense sadness and despair, sudden positivity (this may indicate relief after deciding to follow through on suicide)	Making a will out of the blue	Engaging in risky behavior that could lead to death, such as driving way too fast
Saying goodbye	Researching death or ways to die	Increased drug or alcohol use	Eating or sleeping more or less
Fixation on death or dying	Withdrawing from others	Extreme and sudden mood swings	Saying "I want to die" or "I should kill myself"
Saying things like "I wish I could sleep forever"	Obtaining means, such as pills or a gun or other weapon	Sudden personality changes such as uncharacteristic rage, irritability, anxiety, or agitation	Saying "I wish I were dead" or "I wish I wasn't here"

Table A.3 Do's & Don'ts for Intervention With Suicidal Ideation

Do	Don't
Respond to any statements that include suicidal ideation, even if the person says they are joking.	Be afraid that asking about SI will put the idea in someone's head. This is untrue.

Know that talking about SI removes the taboo and stigma and allows others to talk about it as well.	Assume someone is trying to "get attention." Instead, SI needs attention, and talking about it may be a way to "bring attention."
Sit with them and call 988 – the Suicide and Crisis Lifeline.	Ignore any SI.
Provide resources.	Leave them alone, especially if they have access to lethal means.
Tell them that you care about them.	Tell them to be grateful.
Tell them that you do not want them to die.	Compare their situation to someone else who "has it worse."
Tell them that you want to help.	Keep it a secret.

(Adapted from: https://www.save.org/learn/warning-signs-of-suicide/ and https://supportandsafety. colostate.edu/tell-someone/5-dos-and-donts/)

If you are ever concerned about someone's immediate safety:

- Ensure a safe environment by removing access to means of self-harm.

- Contact emergency services and/or a mental health professional.

- Provide immediate support and actively listen to their concerns.

DOPAMINE AND "DOPAMENUS"

WHY IS DOPAMINE BALANCE IMPORTANT?

Dopamine imbalances affect both mental and physical health. Too much dopamine can lead to aggression and impulsivity, while too little may manifest as depression. Challenges regulating dopamine are linked to conditions like ADHD and addiction.

Physical symptoms include:

- Muscle cramps, spasms, or stiffness

- Digestive issues, such as constipation or reflux

- Pneumonia

- Sleep disturbances

- Slower movement or speech

(Source: HealthDirect)

IDEAS FOR YOUR "DOPAMENU"

Bright light therapy:
Originally used for seasonal affective disorder, this therapy increases dopamine. Sessions typically last 30–90 minutes within the first hour of waking.

Physical activity:
Exercise boosts dopamine and supports overall brain health. Research highlights this bidirectional relationship (Marques et al., 2021).

Specific foods:

1. **Protein-rich foods:** Chicken, turkey, fish, eggs, soy, nuts, and seeds

2. **Fruits/veggies:** Apples, bananas, berries, spinach, kale, avocados

3. **Whole grains:** Oats, quinoa, brown rice

4. **Omega-3s:** Fatty fish, walnuts, flaxseeds

Balancing dopamine is key to emotional regulation, mental health, and physical well-being. Resources like therapy, nutrition, and exercise offer practical tools to support optimal levels.

SUGGESTED DOPAMINE RESOURCES

Video:

- *How to Give Your Brain the Stimulation It Needs* (https://youtu.be/-6WCkTwW6xg?si=YWFRdktih8LdA5F4)

- *How to ADHD* YouTube channel

Books:

- *Dopamine Nation* and *The Official Dopamine Nation Workbook* by Anna Lembke

- *Dopamine for ADHD* by Max Russell

- *How to ADHD: An Insider's Guide to Working With Your Brain (Not Against It)* by Jessica McCabe

Podcast: *ADHD Rewired* (https://www.adhdrewired.com/)

Light boxes: Mayo Clinic. (2022, March 30). *Seasonal affective disorder treatment: Choosing a light box.* https://www.mayoclinic.org/diseases-conditions/seasonal-affective-disorder/in-depth/seasonal-affective-disorder-treatment/art-20048298

MENTAL HEALTH RESOURCES

This comprehensive resource directory connects healthcare professionals to vital mental health resources, including crisis support, therapy, PTSD treatment, grief counseling, and substance abuse services. Programs like the American Nurses Foundation Well-Being Initiative, Emotional PPE Project, and SAMHSA offer free or low-cost aid, ensuring access to essential care for frontline workers.

ACCESS TO SUPPORT, EDUCATION, AND MENTAL HEALTH SERVICES

- American Nurses Foundation Well-Being Initiative: Free mental health tools and resources, including wellness apps for nurses. https://www.nursingworld.org/practice-policy/work-environment/health-safety/disaster-preparedness/coronavirus/what-you-need-to-know/the-well-being-initiative/

- Emotional PPE Project: Free mental health services provided by licensed volunteer clinicians. https://emotionalppe.org/

- Mental Health America: https://mhanational.org/

- NAMI Mental Health Support for Frontline Healthcare Workers: Text "SCRUBS" "HOME" or "FRONTLINE" to 741741

- Therapy Aid Coalition: Free and low-cost short-term therapy for healthcare workers. https://www.therapyaid.org/

- Veterans Crisis Line: https://www.veteranscrisisline.net

DEPRESSION & SUICIDE

- 988 Suicide and Crisis Line: https://988helpline.org/

- National Alliance on Mental Health: https://www.Nami.org

- National Institute of Mental Health: Warning Signs of Suicide. https://www.nimh.nih.gov/health/publications/warning-signs-of-suicide

GRIEF

- A nonprofit organization that offers classes and events to come to your workplace: https://good-grief.org/

- Find your own grief training if it is not offered at your workplace: https://whatsyourgrief.com/supporting-grieving-families-tips-rns-nurses/

- A blog about nurse grief: https://archive.nytimes.com/well.blogs.nytimes.com/2009/04/01/helping-nurses-cope-with-grief/

SUBSTANCE ABUSE

Substance Abuse and Mental Health Services Administration (SAMHSA)—Provides comprehensive information about substance abuse, as well as links to find treatment and other services. https://www.samhsa.gov/find-help/national-helpline

- US Department of Veterans Affairs: National Center for PTSD https://www.ptsd.va.gov/

- Institute of Health: Biometric Telehealth PTSD Treatment Program for Healthcare Workers. https://institutesofhealth.org/ptsd-in-frontline-healthcare-workers/

- Mindful Ethical Clinical Practice and Resilience Academy (MEPRA): A study was conducted showing the efficacy of a 12-week educational program that included "mindfulness, values clarification, self-stewardship, and analytical tools that better prepare healthcare providers for the ethical challenges they often face daily in a hospital setting" (American Association of Critical-Care Nurses, 2023). https://www.aacn.org/newsroom/program-demonstrates-sustained-impact-on-moral-resilience

- https://giving.jhu.edu/story/cynda-rushton-moral-distress/

REFERENCE

Marques, A., Marconcin, P., Werneck, A. O., Ferrari, G., Gouveia, E. R., Kliegel, M., Peralta, M., & Ihle, A. (2021, June 23). Bidirectional association between physical activity and dopamine across adulthood—A systematic review. *Brain Sciences, 11*(7), 829. https://doi.org/10.3390/brainsci11070829

CHAPTER 8

Harnessing the Power of Eustress: The Positive Side of Stress

In a world where stress is often the enemy, *eustress*—a positive form of stress—stands out for its ability to motivate and enhance performance. Unlike distress, which overwhelms and harms well-being, eustress helps us step out of our comfort zones and into growth. It's the adrenaline before a presentation, the excitement of a new challenge, or the anticipation of achieving a goal—stress with a silver lining.

Embracing eustress starts with reframing stressors as opportunities for growth, not threats. This mindset shift allows us to harness eustress to improve focus, cognitive function, and resilience. Research shows that eustress, when balanced correctly, promotes learning, boosts mood, and enhances overall well-being.

The key lies in understanding the differences between eustress and distress:

Eustress (Positive Stress)

1. Motivates goal achievement and personal growth

2. Short-term and manageable

3. Enhances performance, productivity, and focus

4. Promotes positive emotions like excitement and confidence

5. Encourages learning and adaptability

6. Builds resilience for future challenges

Distress (Negative Stress)

1. Overwhelms, causing anxiety or helplessness

2. Chronic and unmanageable

3. Decreases cognitive and physical performance

4. Generates negative emotions like frustration and worry

5. Prevents growth and hinders risk-taking

6. Leads to long-term health issues like heart disease or anxiety disorders

In short, eustress energizes and propels us forward, while distress overwhelms and drains. By embracing eustress, we can thrive and grow in all aspects of life.

CHAPTER 9

AVOIDING IMPOSTER SYNDROME

Imposter syndrome can undermine confidence and performance, especially in high-pressure environments. Recognizing and addressing these feelings is key to overcoming self-doubt, fostering self-acceptance, and embracing success with authenticity.

Here are 10 tips to help avoid imposter syndrome:

1. **Acknowledge your achievements:** Regularly reflect on your successes and the effort that contributed to them. Recognize that your accomplishments are earned.

2. **Reframe negative thoughts:** Challenge self-doubt by replacing it with positive affirmations. Remind yourself that it's okay to make mistakes and grow from them.

3. **Seek support:** Talk to mentors, peers, or friends about your feelings. Chances are that others have experienced similar doubts and can offer reassurance.

4. **Avoid perfectionism:** Understand that perfection is unattainable. Embrace the idea of learning and improving rather than aiming for flawlessness.

5. **Normalize failure:** Accept that everyone fails or makes mistakes. Use setbacks as opportunities for growth rather than signs of inadequacy.

6. **Celebrate small wins:** Recognize and celebrate even the small milestones in your journey. This reinforces your capabilities and boosts confidence.

7. **Focus on your strengths:** Regularly reflect on your skills and talents. Focus on areas where you excel and contribute rather than comparing yourself to others.

8. **Understand that it's common:** Many high-achievers experience imposter syndrome. You're not alone, and it doesn't mean you're incapable.

9. **Stop comparing yourself:** Everyone's journey is unique. Comparison to others often leads to feelings of inadequacy, so focus on your path and progress.

10. **Seek professional help if needed:** If feelings of imposter syndrome are overwhelming, talking to a therapist or counselor can help you address deeper insecurities and build confidence.

Consider enrolling in a Diagnostic Design Thinking Group (https://thinkdifferentlybydesign.com).

INDEX

Note: Page references noted with an *f* are figures; page references noted with a *t* are tables.

J–K

L

M

Q–R

S

T

U

V

W–X

Y–Z

www.ingramcontent.com/pod-product-compliance
Lightning Source LLC
Chambersburg PA
CBHW080421270326
41929CB00018B/3105